Fight Fat, Fight Fatigue
Diet and Cookbook

THE SunSlimmer

Fight Fat, Fight Fatigue
Diet and Cookbook

Sally Ann Voak

Thorsons

VIL 11/02
QY P

Thorsons
An Imprint of HarperCollins*Publishers*
77–85 Fulham Palace Road,
Hammersmith, London W6 8JB

The Thorsons website address is: www.thorsons.com

and *Thorsons*
are trademarks of HarperCollins*Publishers*

Published by Thorsons 2002

10 9 8 7 6 5 4 3 2 1

A catalogue record for this book
is available from the British Library

ISBN 0 00 711869 4

Photography by Steve Lewis

Printed and bound in Great Britain by
Martins the Printers Ltd, Berwick upon Tweed

CONTENTS

For Jan

INTRODUCTION

If you are overweight, and love good food, this is the book for you. It allows you to indulge in the most delicious dishes imaginable, and still lose weight.

It is the third in The Sun Slimmer *Fight Fat, Fight Fatigue* series, which is all about achieving a 'happy weight' while enjoying life to the full – eating well and following exercise routines that are fun, not a chore. The first book, *Energy Makeover*, co-written with GMTV fitness trainer Nicki Waterman, explained the principles of our healthy eating and exercise plan.

In the second volume in the series, *Firm Up All Over,* Nicki went on to provide a whole range of fabulous workouts to help you get into great shape – even if you have only a few minutes to spare.

Now it's my turn to share some of my own discoveries in the field of nutrition and cooking. As Slimming Editor of *The Sun* for the last 30 years, I have learnt that the only way to shape up successfully (and stay in shape after you have achieved your weight and fitness goals) is to have fun while you're doing it. If you feel guilty about every morsel of food you put in your mouth, and mortified when you miss a gruelling session at the gym, you will not succeed. All the people I've interviewed who have managed to keep the weight off for years after successfully following a diet and fitness plan are those who have made substantial changes in their lifestyle and really enjoy their new way of eating and exercising. Interestingly, all of them absolutely love food – and the occasional alcoholic drink.

Personally, I adore messing about in the kitchen, devising new dishes that are healthy as well as tasty. My family are my 'guinea pigs' – particularly my husband, Patrick, who is my greatest critic as well as my most appreciative gourmet 'taster'. Luckily, we both love trying out many different cuisines – from French classical, to Tex-Mex and Eastern, plus, of course, good old British grub. We both now eat more but weigh less than when we married nearly 40 years ago, which must say something about the calorie and fat content of the food I dish up. (And, yes, we do drink alcohol as well, especially wine, beer and our regular evening tipple – whisky and low-calorie ginger ale.)

I hope you have fun trying out my recipes and, of course, following my diet plans. Please write to me (you'll find the address on page 150) and let me know how you get on.

Good luck ... you can do it.

Sally Ann Voak

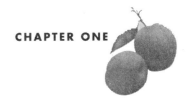

CHAPTER ONE

EAT MORE, WEIGH LESS, BEAT TIREDNESS

Do you feel tired all the time? Are you trapped in a constant round of yo-yo dieting – losing weight, then regaining it, plus a little bit more? Do you join a slimming club then get bored with the diet and use lame excuses to stop going to club meetings? Are you so tired by lunchtime that you pig out on high-fat food just to keep yourself going?

If any of the above sound familiar, take heart. You are not a slimming failure. You are simply suffering from a kind of starvation. Yes, despite all those attempts to shape up, you are actually depriving yourself of the vital nourishment your body desperately needs to fight disease and keep you in good shape. Like many people, you probably try hard to 'be good' – skipping breakfast, fighting hunger pangs, feeling guilty every time you look at a chocolate. Not surprisingly, you find it hard to keep up the effort for more than a few months, and drift back into your 'bad' old eating habits.

Let's get one thing straight, there is nothing 'bad' about food. In *Energy Makeover*, the first book in this series, I explained how eating regular, nourishing, filling meals is the key to permanent weight loss. This book expands on that theory by giving practical guidance on how to plan your meals and cook fabulous dishes that will make you feel, and look, just great.

TIREDNESS AND BEING OVERWEIGHT –
WHY ARE THEY CONNECTED?

Are you getting enough? Food, that is. You probably think you are already eating far too much and should cut down. NO! The problem is that you are eating the wrong things, at the wrong time and there is probably not enough variety in your diet either. Compare yourself to a car. You need 'fuel' in the form of food and drink to keep your body running smoothly. Just as there is no point in filling up your petrol tank before you put the car into the garage, there is no point in eating a huge, fat-laden meal just before you go to bed.

Similarly, after 12 hours of fasting during the night, your 'tank' needs filling again. And, of course, if you use good quality 'fuel' (i.e. lots of varied, delicious foods instead of the same old burgers and chips) your body will run much more smoothly. Instead of looking like a rusty old banger, you'll look and feel like a sports model. OK, sorry about the clichés, but it's true.

You're bound to have read newspaper and magazine articles that list all the nutrients that are supplied by food, and how much we need. As a brief reminder, the principal nutrients are protein, fat and carbohydrate. These days, adults usually get enough protein (in foods like meat, fish, beans), far too much fat (in fast food like burgers and Chinese takeaways, and 'hidden' in processed foods, biscuits, cakes and puddings), and not enough good quality carbohydrate (in high-fibre foods such as fruit, vegetables, cereals and bread).

If you look at the plate on page 4 you will see what your daily diet should be made up of. As you can see, most of your daily intake should be carbohydrates – fruit, vegetables, potatoes, cereals, breads, grains. Carbs have had a bit of a bad press recently, so you may be wondering if you can still eat plenty when you're trying to lose weight. The answer is definitely YES. Carbs are still winners. Carb-rich foods are lower in calories and more filling than fatty foods, so it makes sense to tuck in. Believe me, the new crop of diets which exclude carbs and rely on protein and high-fat foods to help you slim are dangerous: they overwork the kidneys, cause constipation and bad breath and can even contribute to heart disease by 'furring up' the arteries. I am now getting a stream of letters from slimmers who have shed weight on these diets, but are scared to re-introduce carbohydrate into their diets for fear of fattening up. A lifetime of eating steak and lettuce is not a happy prospect.

It's also wise to be aware of the GI factor. The GI or glycaemic index is a ranking of foods from 1 to 100 based on the rate at which each food raises the blood sugar level. Foods with a low GI factor (wholemeal bread, fruit, vegetables etc.) cause a slow rise, while foods with a high GI factor (cakes, sweets etc.) cause a rapid rise, which can then cause a dip in blood sugar, and lead to hunger. However, this effect can change when other foods are eaten at the same time (a piece of wholemeal bread spread with butter, for instance), so it can be confusing. The best way to ensure that your blood sugar level is kept on an even keel is to eat regular meals and sensible low-fat, high-carb snacks between them.

Eat More, Weigh Less, Beat Tiredness

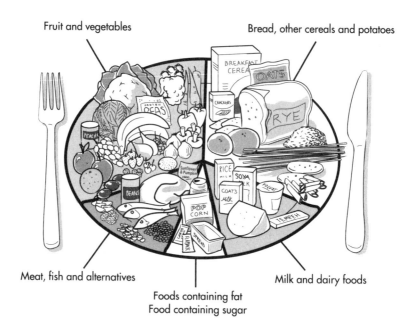

Fruit and vegetables

Bread, other cereals and potatoes

Meat, fish and alternatives

Foods containing fat
Food containing sugar

Milk and dairy foods

As well as carbs, protein and fat, we also need the various vitamins and minerals that are found in natural foods. These are vital for good health and to prevent disease. A number of very important vitamins and minerals cannot be stored by the body, so a daily intake is needed. For instance, vitamin C (found in fruit and vegetables) – which is essential for healthy skin, iron absorption, wound healing and resistance to infection – needs 'topping up' regularly. So too does iron (found in meat, wholegrain cereals), as it forms part of the haemoglobin in red blood cells that carry oxygen to all parts of the body. It's estimated that one in three women of child-bearing age in this country is iron deficient. Vitamins and minerals can also be lost in cooking, so there really is a very good reason to improve your cooking skills, and add variety to your diet.

Is all booze bad for you? Alcohol makes you tired, dehydrated, fuddles your brain and makes you fat. Ah, yes, but isn't it lovely? I would be the last person to say that you have to cut out drinking if you want to slim. However, the hard facts are that it is high in calories (about 100 for a half pint of beer or glass of wine), has a depressant effect on the brain and central nervous system, and stimulates the gastric juices.

So, if you drink before a meal, you will find that you are less able to make a sensible choice about what you are eating. You will also feel hungrier when you sit down at the table. Booze also dehydrates the whole body, which accounts for the dry skin and red eyeballs that greet you when you look in the mirror after a bender. Women break down alcohol at a slower rate than men, which is unfair but worth remembering if you are a driver. As a lover of good wine and Guinness, I have to say that I now know what I wish I'd known at the age of 25: booze is OK in small doses and you should match each glass of wine with an equal quantity of water. Enough said.

To slim successfully, therefore, we need to do three things:

1. Lower our calorie and fat intake, while eating a wide variety of good foods – including at least five portions of fruit and vegetables each day.

2. Eat regularly, so we don't experience those awful between-meals cravings that can lead to chronic tiredness and binge-eating.

3. Find a diet which has so many good things to eat that we want to follow the same kind of eating plan...for life.

I think you will find that this book will give you all of the above, and a lot of enjoyment as well.

Eat More, Weigh Less, Beat Tiredness

HOW TO USE THIS BOOK

I've divided the book into two sections: The Diets and The Recipes. At the end of the book (page 149) is a list of handy websites and addresses which will help you add to your knowledge about healthy eating and nutrition. Here's what the two main sections contain:

The Diets

This section of the book has five great versions of my original Fight Fat, Fight Fatigue Diet Plan. Each one contains easy meals, many of which can be prepared using recipes from the second half of the book (these recipes have a page reference, so you'll know where to find them).

The Quick Weight-loss Diet is very effective if you need to shed up to half a stone in a hurry: for instance, if you are going on holiday or want to get into shape for a special occasion. It is safe, easy to follow and works quickly. This plan can also be used to 'kick start' your slimming programme, or to 'shake up' your metabolism if you just can't shed any more weight on your current eating programme.

Lose Three Stone is a plan for women or men who have three stone or more to shed. Again, it is very simple to follow. You can follow it safely for as long as you need to reach your goal. However, with such a lot of weight to lose, I suggest you take it easy, aiming for half a stone, then another half-stone and so on. The foods are delicious, you can eat out if you like, and yes, you can have a drink or two!

For Men Only is aimed at blokes with beer bellies. Sorry to be a bit basic, but if you have one (even if it wasn't caused by beer), you'll know what I mean. If you've found the weight creeping on over the years, yet you still want to enjoy good food and the occasional night out at the pub you'll enjoy this diet. It has lots of hints and tips especially suited to men, and the meals are hearty and filling.

Teen Eating Plan is just what it says – a healthy eating plan for 13 to 19 year olds who want to get fit and slim. No, I don't apologize for suggesting that youngsters should be encouraged and shown how to eat healthily. I am convinced that lack of knowledge is one reason why many kids get eating disorders. My plan gives them the facts.

How to Maintain Your Weight Loss is a no-fail diet plan which, if you follow it properly, will ensure that all your good efforts are rewarded – with a slim-line future. You can adjust your own calorie intake to suit yourself so your weight remains fairly steady throughout your life.

7

THE RECIPES

I have divided this section of the book into six parts, each containing 10–12 great recipes. Unless otherwise stated, all quantities are for four people, and I give the calorie and fat content per serving. At the end of most recipes are 'Nutrition Notes' that explain which nutrients (vitamins, minerals etc.) are in the dish concerned, and what they can do for you. The six sections are as follows:

Brilliant Breakfasts are easy to prepare, yet contain all the goodness you need to make you feel energetic until lunchtime. They include some unusual things as well. You might not have thought of dishing up my Harem Breakfast (almonds, oranges, dates, cottage cheese) to your beloved on a Sunday morning, but, believe me, it works wonders.

Scrummy Snacks and Nibbles are my energy boosters which can be used pre- or post-exercise or just between meals when you're feeling droopy. They include things like Italian Bruschetta with Parmesan, Microwaved Bananas with Cinnamon, and a whole range of ideas on what to add to crispbreads and rice cakes.

Perfect Packed Lunches are so tasty that you'll wonder why you've ever paid a fortune for a dried-up sandwich when, with a little planning, you could have enjoyed a feast. I recommend the Chicken and Ham Pâté with Oriental Salad for a picnic, and the Bean and Vegetable Soup is the most comforting, filling midday 'snack' I've ever tasted.

Family Supper Dishes will end forever the cry of 'boooooooring' that goes up when a parent suggests a healthy meal. These may be healthy, but boring they ain't. I defy any teenager not to approve of Chicken Maryland, while Pancakes with Ricotta Cheese and Spinach will win approval from the vegetarians of the family.

Dinner Party Dishes are designed to fool your supper guests into thinking they are visiting a telly chef. With absolutely the minimum of effort, you will stun them with your Borscht with Caviar followed by Ginger Beef Steaks with Pineapple Salsa.

Picnics and Barbecues shows you how to fill up hungry people without fattening them up as well. With the simplest ingredients you can make meals that are easy to pack up and serve as a picnic, or quick to cook on the barbie. Most of the recipes can be used indoors too.

Ready to eat yourself slim? Go for it.

THE DIETS

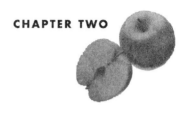

CHAPTER TWO

THE QUICK WEIGHT-LOSS DIET

Lose up to half a stone in three weeks

The Fight Fat, Fight Fatigue diet is a life-long healthy eating programme which helps you change your body shape and fitness level over a period of three months or more. However, there are times when a more rapid weight loss is required, so here is the diet plan that can do the job safely.

There are all kinds of reasons why you may need it. For instance, you may be planning a holiday next month and need to 'fine-tune' your body so you look and feel your best on the beach. You may have just returned from a trip, and discovered that you weigh a few pounds more than you did before you went.

Other times when you need this plan include that period of re-adjustment after a life-change such as a new job, a house move or wedding. With the best will in the world, you may have tried hard to stick with your fitness and eating programme, but somehow high-fat food and extra alcohol has crept into your life. The result: your exercise routine flies out of the window and you feel lumpy and frumpy.

Fear not, you WILL recover, and this three-week programme will help you do it. I have made this diet the most nutritious and interesting plan I can devise, within the scope of a daily 1500 calorie limit and a nutritional balance of about 50 per cent carbohydrate, 30 per cent fat, 20 per cent protein. The carbs are reasonably high because I want you to combine the diet with exercise – following a suitable programme in Nicki Waterman's book, *Firm Up All Over*. Carbs are needed to fuel your muscles for exercise so don't restrict them.

Because it is important to follow this diet exactly, you must plan ahead. Read the diet through, go shopping for the foods you need each week, and keep a daily 'food diary' of exactly what you have eaten. Writing it down will help you stick to it. Take a packed lunch to work if possible, so you are in control.

Follow the diet for three weeks. You will see that many of the meal suggestions use recipes from this book, so this is a good opportunity for you to try them. There's even a booze allowance and meal choices for a night out on the town. Enjoy!

DIET PLAN

This plan is suitable for people who are less than 3st overweight. It contains about 1500 calories daily, is low in fat and high in vitamins and minerals. If you are vegetarian, there are lots of meal choices for you. Men can follow it too, but should add 100g/4oz lean meat, fish or Quorn daily, plus an extra 200g/7oz of potato, pasta or rice.

Daily Allowances

MILK
½ pint semi-skimmed milk for tea, coffee and to pour on cereals.

BOOZE
½ pint lager or 1 glass dry wine daily. Men can have an extra ½ pint lager or glass of wine. If you wish, save up your booze allowance for weekends. Drink plenty of water – about 3 litres daily.

FREE VEGETABLES
You can eat as much as you like from the following list of very low-calorie vegetables: asparagus, beansprouts, broccoli, Brussels sprouts, cabbage, cauliflower, celery, lettuce, mushrooms, mustard and cress, pak choi, peppers (red, green, yellow), radishes, runner beans, spinach, spring onions, tomatoes (canned and fresh), watercress, water chestnuts. Cook your vegetables lightly, or as a stir-fry (instead of using fat use a little water), and serve salads with a lemon juice and herb dressing or a tablespoon of fat-free vinaigrette dressing.

HERBS, SPICES AND SAUCES
You can also have as much as you like from the following list: freshly ground black pepper, garlic, ginger, allspice, curry powder, Chinese five spice sauce, light soy sauce, Worcestershire sauce, oriental fish sauce, lemon and lime juice.

Important: do not add salt in cooking, or sprinkle it on food.

The Quick Weight-loss Diet

13

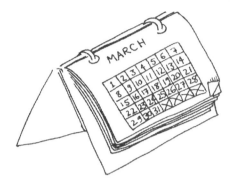

WEEK ONE

You will lose most weight this week – up to about 2–4lbs. But don't forget that a lot of this is water. It is important not to skip meals, and to eat the snacks and nibbles where included. If you are exercising regularly (and you should be), you can also have a 'diet extra'. This should be used as a 'recovery' food after your workout, accompanied by several glasses of water.

BREAKFASTS (Choose One)

- Harem Breakfast (see recipe, page 69), 1 slice wholemeal toast with jam or marmalade, small glass fruit juice
- Medium portion Special K or 1 Weetabix, milk from allowance, small sliced banana, small glass fruit juice
- Fruit Smoothie (see recipe, page 75), 1 slice wholemeal toast with jam or marmalade
- Scrambled Egg with Mushrooms (see recipe, page 67), 1 slice wholemeal toast, small glass orange juice
- 1 slice toast topped with 1 rasher well-grilled back bacon, watercress, grilled tomatoes (as many as you like) and mushrooms poached in stock or water, small glass fruit juice
- Sandwich of 2 thin slices wholemeal bread, salad, 1 rasher well-grilled back bacon, crumbled
- Half small melon, seeded, chopped, mixed with 1 tbsp muesli and some sliced fresh nectarine, and 1 small carton diet yogurt poured over the top; small glass fruit juice

15

MID-MORNING (Choose One)

- Any Rice Cake or Crispbread Topper (see list, page 85)

LUNCHES (Choose One)

- Low-Fat Hummus with Pitta and Salad (see recipe, page 101), 1 apple, orange or small banana, diet soft drink
- 2 slices wholemeal bread spread with mild mustard or a scraping of low-fat cheese spread with one of these fillings: 50g/2oz any lean meat; 100g/4oz fish canned in tomato sauce, brine or water (eg. tuna, mackerel); 25g/1oz grated hard cheese; 100g/4oz cottage cheese. Plus: 1 apple, orange, small banana, or small bunch grapes
- 250g/10oz jacket potato served with a huge mixed salad and one of these toppings: 3 tbsp baked beans, 100g/4oz tuna mashed with lemon juice and pepper, 2 tbsp salsa dip with 1 tbsp grated Parmesan cheese. Plus: 1 orange or kiwi fruit
- Stuffed Peppers with Creamy Coleslaw (See recipe, page 96)

MID-AFTERNOON (Choose One)

- 6 dried apricots
- 1 apple and 1 kiwi fruit
- Small carton diet yogurt (any flavour) with 1 pear or nectarine.

SUPPERS (Choose One)

- Lower-fat Oriental Stir-fry (see recipe, page 110), 4 tbsp boiled rice or noodles, huge mixed side salad (chosen from 'free' vegetable list), small banana or small wholemeal roll

Fight Fat, Fight Fatigue Diet and Cookbook

- Lean grilled beefburger or Quorn Quarterpounder, vegetables from 'free' list, 200g/8oz jacket potato, low-fat fromage frais with sliced peach or nectarine
- Leek and Seafood Lasagne (see recipe, page 112), large mixed salad, individual meringue base topped with sliced kiwi fruit and squirt of aerosol cream
- 250g/10oz grilled chicken breast (no skin), grilled tomatoes, mushrooms poached in stock, green vegetables from 'free' list, 4 tbsp boiled brown rice or cooked wholemeal pasta, and 1 apple, orange or pear
- Large slice melon with ginger, 200g/8oz grilled trout or mackerel with lemon juice, 100g/4oz oven chips, vegetables and salad from 'free' list, small wholemeal roll, baked apple with 1 tsp honey and 1 tbsp raisins and 1 tsp natural yogurt poured over
- 50g/2oz any lean roast meat or veggie equivalent, thin gravy, huge portion of 'free' vegetables, 75g/3oz chunk dry-roast potato (par-boil, then brush lightly with oil and crisp under the grill), small portion Filo-topped Fruit Pie (see recipe, page 131)
- Restaurant meal: Indian meal of chicken shaslik or tikka, salad, plain boiled rice; or Italian meal of seafood salad, pasta with tomatoes

DIET EXTRAS (Choose one as a post-exercise booster with plenty of water to drink)

- Medium banana
- Crispbread topped with Aubergine Pâté with Garlic (see recipe, page 81)
- Bruschetta with Parmesan (see recipe, page 82)
- 1 small carton diet yogurt (any flavour), 1 apple
- Special K bar

The Quick Weight-loss Diet

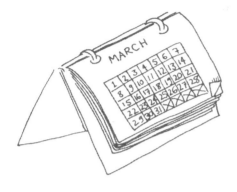

WEEK TWO

Well done! You now realize that 'going back to the drawing board' really does work. This week there are more delicious meals and snacks to try, and you should 'up' your exercise level as well. That means more walking, cycling or swimming. And don't forget those pre-workout stretching exercises.

BREAKFASTS (Choose One)

- Large bowl any cereal, milk from allowance, sliced apple, 2 tbsp low-fat natural yogurt
- 2 slices wholemeal toast with Marmite and grilled or cold tomatoes, small glass fruit juice
- 50g/2oz porridge oats made with water, milk from allowance, small carton diet yogurt, 1 tsp honey, small glass fruit juice
- Scrambled Egg with Mushrooms (see recipe, page 67), 1 slice wholemeal toast
- Apple and Lime Crunchie (see recipe, page 68), digestive biscuit for dunking
- Sandwich of 2 thin slices wholemeal bread, 1 tsp jam, 1 small mashed banana
- Fresh fruit salad made from chunks of melon, frozen raspberries, sliced apple, small sliced banana, 2 tbsp natural yogurt; 1 crispbread spread with 1 tsp jam or marmalade

MID-MORNING (Choose One)

- 2 jaffa cakes
- 1 crispbread topped with 2 tsp low-fat soft cheese, tomatoes and watercress
- Packet of low-fat crisps or Quavers
- 1 orange and 1 apple

LUNCHES (Choose One)

- Curried Chicken Breasts with Spicy Carrot Dip (see recipe, page 94)
- Wholemeal pitta bread or tortilla wrap stuffed with salad and one of these fillings: Aubergine Pâté with Garlic (see recipe, page 81); 50g/2oz cold cooked chicken, turkey or lean pork, no skin; 100g/4oz tuna or salmon canned in brine, with lots of lemon juice and pepper. Plus 2 plums, or small bunch grapes, or 1 pear or nectarine
- Bean and Vegetable Soup (see recipe, page 93), small crusty roll, kiwi fruit
- Any high street sandwich, pitta or flatbread containing 300 calories or less. Plus apple, small banana, pear or orange
- 100g/4oz any cold meat, fish or Quorn dish with large mixed salad from 'free' list, 200g/8oz jacket potato
- Italian Rice Salad (see recipe, page 88), small wholemeal roll spread with 2 tsp low-fat cheese spread, medium banana

MID-AFTERNOON (Choose One)

- 1 apple with 25g/1oz raisins or 3 dried apricots
- Small banana
- Mug of Ovaltine Options and 1 jaffa cake
- 2 crispbreads spread with lemon curd
- Small carton diet yogurt (any flavour)

SUPPERS (Choose One)

- Ginger Beef Steak with Pineapple Salsa (see recipe, page 126), 4 tbsp boiled brown rice or noodles, 125g/4oz low-fat fromage frais with sliced peach or nectarine
- Normandy Pork (see recipe, page 109), 75g/3oz mashed potato (use skimmed milk for mashing), large portion 'free' vegetables, small carton of diet yogurt (any flavour)
- Any rice or pasta-based supermarket ready-meal of 400 calories or less, plus lots of 'free' vegetables and salad
- Large slice melon with ginger, 50g/2oz lean roast meat or veggie equivalent, thin gravy, large portion 'free' vegetables, Chocolate Mousse with Rum (see recipe, page 133)
- 250g/10oz grilled mackerel, sardines or other oily fish, with lemon, garlic and herbs. Plus Chinese Salad with Ginger (see recipe, page 147), 1 orange or pear
- Eating Out: carvery meal of melon, followed by lean meat, 'free' vegetables, 1 scoop vanilla ice-cream; or bistro meal of crudités (mixed raw vegetables) or moules marinières (mussels cooked in wine and cream) with grilled steak or fish and salad to follow

21

DIET EXTRAS (Choose one as a post-exercise booster with plenty of water to drink)

- Any Meringue Nest Topper (see recipes, page 86)
- Microwaved Banana with Cinnamon (see recipe, page 87)
- Small bowl any cereal with milk from allowance

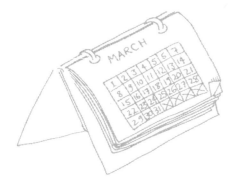

WEEK THREE

Go for it! This is the countdown week which will end with a glorious victory. If you have been following the diet properly, you will have lost at least half a stone by the end of the next seven days – and eaten all this delicious food as well. Wow.

BREAKFASTS (Choose One)

- Medium bowl any cereal, milk from allowance, small sliced banana, small glass fruit juice
- Harem Breakfast (see recipe, page 69), 1 slice wholemeal toast, a few grapes
- Egg and Bacon Soufflé Omelette (see recipe, page 73), small glass fruit juice
- Medium boiled egg, 1 slice wholemeal toast, medium glass fruit juice
- 1 Weetabix, milk from allowance, sliced pear, 2 tbsp natural unsweetened yogurt or low-fat fromage frais, medium glass fruit juice
- Sandwich of 2 thin slices wholemeal bread, 1 rasher well-grilled back bacon, tomatoes, watercress

23

MID-MORNING (Choose One)

- Packet of low-fat crisps
- 2 crispbreads with 2 tsp low-fat soft cheese, cucumber, watercress, tomatoes
- 1 apple and 3 dried apricots
- 2 jaffa cakes

LUNCHES (Choose One)

- Sandwich of 2 slices wholemeal bread spread with mild mustard or Marmite, plus salad and one of these fillings: 2 Quorn slices, sliced hard-boiled egg, 4 sardines canned in tomato sauce or brine, 50g/2oz lean cold ham or other cooked meat. Plus small bunch grapes, pear, peach or nectarine, or 8 strawberries or raspberries

MID-AFTERNOON (Choose One)

- 2 jaffa cakes
- Small banana
- 2 crispbreads with Smoked Mackerel Pâté (see recipe, page 89)
- 1 apple and 1 pear

SUPPERS (Choose One)

- Chicken Maryland (see recipe, page 106), large portion of 'free' vegetables and salad
- Mixed Stuffed Vegetables (see recipe, page 114), large mixed salad from 'free' list
- Plaice with Mustard Sauce (see recipe, page 115), 100g/4oz oven chips or 250g/10oz jacket potato, vegetables and salad from 'free' list
- Pears Roquefort (see recipe, page 125), 50g/2oz any lean roast meat or veggie equivalent, thin gravy, vegetables from 'free' list

- Slice of melon, Mexican Baked Trout (see recipe, page 130); mixed salad, 125g/4oz low-fat fromage frais with small, sliced banana
- Well-grilled beefburger or Quorn Quarterpounder, grilled tomatoes, watercress, 200g/8oz jacket potato, huge mixed salad, large bowl fresh or frozen raspberries or blackberries with 2 tbsp low-fat natural yogurt
- Any rice- or pasta-based ready-meal of under 400 calories, 'free' salad and vegetables

DIET EXTRAS (Choose one as a post-exercise booster with plenty of water to drink)

- Small bowl cereal with a few raisins on top, and milk from allowance
- Small banana
- 2 crispbreads topped with 2 tsp jam and sliced kiwi fruit
- Special K bar

25

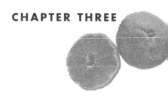

CHAPTER THREE

LOSE THREE STONE

When you've got a big weight on your mind...

Sounds daunting, doesn't it? Forty-two pounds of excess flab to shed. That could mean a whole year of calorie counting, meagre meals and alcohol deprivation. Yuk!

It doesn't have to be like that. With our Fight Fat, Fight Fatigue eating programme, there is no calorie counting, no deprivation (the meals are enormous, the snacks are filling and you can enjoy some booze) – and no boredom. Here's how this version of the diet can work for you. Suppose, for example, that you now weigh 13st and would like to weigh

10st, or weigh 15st and would like to weigh 12st. Maybe you have already spent a good few years 'yo-yo-ing' – losing a few pounds, or stones, then regaining them, and more?

Frankly, any attempt to crash diet would now inevitably end up with a weight GAIN. That's because your body is now totally fed up with all this messing around and will be prompted, via the appetite centres of your brain, to store energy whenever it gets the chance. So, once you stop following that drastic diet plan, you will balloon.

There is a better way. With the diet plan below, you will re-educate yourself (both brain and body) to eat properly. It will not be a chore, because the meals are enjoyable, and there is no calorie counting necessary. It will not be boring, because there is a huge variety of food to choose from, and you certainly can have some alcohol – every day if you like.

Will it still take a year to shed that three stone? Who knows? We are all different. If you are young, active and determined, it could take three months. If you are older and have spent years skipping from one club diet to another, but taken very little exercise, it will take longer to revitalize your poor old nutrient- and activity-starved body.

The best line of attack is to give yourself a 7lb weight-loss target. Once you've shed that amount (the equivalent of 7 full cans of tomato soup or 3 kilos of new potatoes), set yourself another half-stone target, and so on. Every time you reach a target, reward yourself with an outing: to the shops, the cinema, the seaside, depending on your inclination and budget. You should also write down everything you eat in a 'food diary' – this makes you think very hard about what you are eating and helps you stick to the programme.

The best thing about this diet plan is that it makes you feel a whole lot more energetic. So, to burn off this energy (and your excess flab), make sure you embark on an exercise programme as well – one such as Nicki Waterman's *Firm Up All Over.*

Before you start, look at your lifestyle. The hard truth is that someone who slims down but does not make changes in their lifestyle at the same time is very likely to regain the weight they lose. I am not just talking about taking more exercise (although that is very important), but also changing your 'mind-set'. Make a list of everything you are doing now, and another one itemizing everything you want to achieve. Take positive steps to change things so that your life becomes more like the second list. Whether that means learning new skills, meeting new friends, or dyeing your hair blond (or all three), give it a try. You will only become the slim, confident person of your dreams if you recognize that you must improve the whole package – not just the wrapping.

DIET PLAN

This plan is for people who want to shed about 3st. It contains about 1650 calories daily, is low in fat and high in vitamins and minerals. If you are vegetarian, there are plenty of meal choices. Men should add 150g/6oz lean meat, fish or Quorn daily, plus 250g/10oz potato or 150g/6oz pasta or rice.

It is very important that you eat everything on the diet. One of the best ways to rev up your sluggish metabolism is to start each day with a good breakfast – so make sure you eat one of the choices below. No excuses ...

Daily Allowances

MILK

Your daily milk allowance is ½ pint semi-skimmed for tea, coffee and to pour on cereals.

BOOZE

½ pint lager, 1 glass dry wine or 2 pub-measure 'short' drinks with low-calorie mixers only. (Remember that we tend to serve up doubles at home!). Men can have an extra ½ pint lager, glass of wine or short drink with low-calorie mixers.

FREE VEGETABLES

You can eat as much as you like from the following list of very low-calorie vegetables: asparagus, beansprouts, broccoli, Brussels sprouts, cabbage, cauliflower, celery, lettuce, mushrooms, mustard and cress, pak choi, peppers (red, green, yellow), radishes, runner beans, spinach, spring onions, tomatoes (canned and fresh), watercress, water chestnuts. Cook your vegetables lightly, or as a stir-fry (use a little water instead of oil or use little oil and a few tablespoons of water).

Make sure your salads are huge, and imaginative – use spinach leaves, grated carrot and cauliflower florets as well as the traditional lettuce, tomatoes and cucumber. You need those vitamins and minerals. Serve salads with a lemon juice and herb dressing or a tablespoon of fat-free vinaigrette dressing.

HERBS, SPICES AND SAUCES

You can also have as much as you like from the following list: freshly ground black pepper, garlic, ginger, allspice, curry powder, Chinese five spice sauce, light soy sauce, Worcestershire sauce, oriental fish sauce, lemon and lime juice.

EVERY DAY choose one breakfast, one lunch, one supper, two snacks and one 'diet extra' from the lists below. The diet extra choices are meant to boost your nutrition for exercise, so eat them an hour or so before you exercise.

BREAKFASTS

- Egg and Bacon Soufflé Omelette (see recipe, page 73), 2 crispbreads with a little low-fat spread, small glass fruit juice
- 2 Weetabix or medium bowl any cereal (use a Kellogg's Variety Pack, so you can ring the changes), milk from allowance, slice of wholemeal toast with 2 tsp jam or marmalade, small glass fruit juice
- 2 slices wholemeal toast topped with poached egg, watercress, grilled tomatoes, 1 apple
- 2 eggs, scrambled with sliced mushrooms, 1 tbsp sweetcorn and milk from allowance; watercress, grilled tomatoes, 1 thin slice wholemeal toast, small glass fruit juice
- 30g/1½ oz porridge made up with water, topped with milk from allowance, medium sliced banana and apple or kiwi fruit and a few raisins
- Apricot and Banana Compote (see recipe, page 98 – save some for lunch tomorrow!), slice of wholemeal toast with 1 tsp jam or marmalade
- Sandwich of 2 slices wholemeal bread, with one of the following fillings: sliced boiled egg, watercress, tomatoes; 1 rasher well-grilled back bacon, cucumber, tomatoes, mustard; small, sliced banana, 1 tbsp low-fat Greek yogurt; 2 thin slices corned beef or leftover cooked chicken (no skin), mustard, grated carrot, sliced celery, watercress. Plus 1 apple or pear
- Boiled egg, slice of wholemeal toast with low-fat spread, medium glass fruit juice, and 1 apple, orange, pear or peach

- Fresh fruit salad: slice 1 apple, 1 peach, top with strawberries or raspberries and 1 small carton any flavour diet yogurt. Sprinkle 1 tbsp mixed nuts on top and use a small digestive biscuit for dunking

LUNCHES

- 200g/8oz cooked chicken (no skin), 'free' salad, Apricot and Banana Compote (see recipe, page 98)
- Any 300-calorie high street sandwich, flatbread, roll or stuffed pitta; plus 1 apple, orange, pear, peach or nectarine
- Stuffed Peppers with Creamy Coleslaw (see recipe, page 96), huge salad from 'free' list, small wholemeal roll with scraping of low-fat spread
- 2 slices wholemeal bread or medium wholemeal roll with salad and one of these fillings: Aubergine Pâté with Garlic (see recipe, page 81) or 2 tsp low fat cheese spread, 50g/2oz lean meat or 100g/4oz tuna or salmon canned in brine. Plus small carton diet yogurt and a few grapes or 3 dried apricots
- Low-fat Hummus with Pitta and Salad (see recipe, page 101), small banana
- 175g/6oz any oily fish (eg. trout, mackerel, sardines) grilled with garlic and lemon juice, large mixed salad and vegetables from 'free' list, slice of wholemeal bread, kiwi fruit or orange
- Quorn Quarterpounder, grilled, with grilled tomatoes and mushrooms, salad and vegetables from 'free' list; small carton diet yogurt or fromage frais with large portion strawberries or raspberries
- 250g/10oz jacket potato, split and served with a large mixed salad from 'free' list and topped with 3 tbsp baked beans or 100g/4oz tuna, canned in brine, mashed with lemon juice and pepper

SUPPERS

- Large slice melon with ginger, Normandy Pork (see recipe, page 109), 75g/3oz mashed potato (use milk from allowance for mashing), 'free' vegetables, slice of wholemeal bread
- Beef Casserole with Guinness (see recipe, page 118), 75g/3oz mashed potato (use milk from allowance for mashing), 'free' vegetables, medium banana
- Filo Surprise Parcels (see recipe, page 129), large salad from 'free' list, Chocolate Mousse with Rum (see recipe, page 133) or 1 carton crème caramel
- Any rice- or pasta-based ready meal of 400 calories, plenty of 'free' vegetables and salad, plus apple and pear or nectarine and kiwi fruit
- 50g/2oz any lean roast meat, vegetarian nut roast or Quorn roast; thin gravy, 75g/3oz chunk roast potato, plenty of 'free' vegetables, Slimmers' Pavlova (see recipe, page 132)
- Mixed Stuffed Vegetables (see recipe, page 114), large mixed salad, small carton low-fat fromage frais or low-fat yogurt
- 175g/6oz any oily fish (eg. mackerel, salmon, herrings) grilled with lemon juice and garlic or other herbs, 200g/8oz jacket potato, 'free' vegetables, baked apple with 2 tbsp low-fat yogurt or fromage frais, 1 tsp honey, 2 tsp raisins
- Small can slimmer's soup (any flavour), 150g/5oz lean lamb chop, pork tenderloin or Quorn Quarterpounder, grilled with rosemary and garlic, 75g/3oz potato, mashed with semi-skimmed milk and Dijon mustard to taste, 'free' vegetables, small crusty roll
- Eating out: carvery meal of lean meat or grilled fish with plenty of 'free' vegetables, 2 scoops vanilla ice-cream, 1 wafer. Or Indian meal of Chicken Tikka or Tandoori or Chicken or Prawn Shaslik, salad, 3 tbsp plain boiled rice, 1 poppadum. Or Italian meal of melon with parma ham, pasta with tomato or vongole (clam) sauce, large mixed salad

SNACKS

- Rice Cake or Crispbread Topper (see list, page 85), satsuma or a few grapes
- Meringue Nest Topper (see list, page 86)
- Slice of toast with 1 tsp jam or lemon curd
- 1 apple and 1 pear or nectarine
- Medium banana

DIET EXTRAS

- 2 fingers Kit Kat or 1 fun-size choc bar
- 1 packet low-fat crisps
- Extra half-pint stout or beer

33

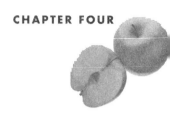

CHAPTER FOUR

FOR MEN ONLY

How to lose that beer belly

If you are a bloke who is trying to improve his health and well-being by shaping up, then good for you. Although it may not be very cool to admit that you are 'on a diet', these days most men do feel comfortable telling their friends that they are trying to eat more healthily and take more exercise.

For many overweight men the crunch comes when they go to visit their doctor with a nagging problem such as backache, breathlessness or tiredness and are told that 'it might be a good idea to shed some of that excess baggage'. Those few words can concentrate the mind very swiftly. But how do you do it? Well there is no need to starve yourself, or deprive yourself of the odd pint or glass of wine. All you have to do is follow my diet plan.

Perhaps you only need to shed a stone or two? Maybe you have a wobbly tum, and even a wobbly bum as well? If your weight has crept up over the years (or piled on since you gave up playing sports), now is the time to act. Follow the plan until you reach your ideal weight and shape. To help improve your general fitness, try to include at least 20 minutes of cardio-vascular exercise (brisk walking, treadmill, bike-riding etc.) every day.

If you need to shed three stone or more, you are right to be worried about your excess flab. It is well documented that being very overweight is dangerous: it can increase your chances of succumbing to heart disease, diabetes, cancer and other serious health problems. Have a fitness check-up before you start my diet (it is important to find out, for instance, if you are diabetic – in which case, you will be given a diet plan by your doctor).

If you have a partner who is also overweight, they can follow one of the plans in the diet section of the book. As you will see, many of the recipes are the same for men and women, so it is easy to slim together.

35

Here are my ten top tips for men who want to shed weight:

1. Be in control. If you are in a job which involves lots of driving, buy a coolbox so you take your lunch, mineral water and snack foods with you. Don't be tempted to stray into motorway services for a greasy, overpriced meal or stock up with chocs at petrol stations.

2. Don't build your social life around the pub. If you have drifted into the habit of having a few bevvies after work, go to the gym or swimming pool instead. Think of the hours you spend boozing. Life is too short. Although a convivial drink is terrific, there are other things to do as well, such as playing sports, going to the cinema, concerts, the theatre...

3. Improve your cooking skills. A man who is a whizz in the kitchen is likely to be equally talented in bed. Think about it: a bloke who can make a beautiful salad, dish up a roast with finesse, or create an aphrodisiac meal for two obviously has the imagination and skills to be good at other things as well!

4. Reward yourself for your efforts with some new clothes, aftershave, haircut. As the weight drops off, you will feel proud of your shape.

5. Take more exercise. If you don't have any health problems that prevent you exercising, start off with some brisk walking and swimming. Then join a good gym, have a fitness assessment and start a properly organized training schedule. These days, gyms are full of guys of all ages, shapes and sizes, so there is no need to feel embarrassed. Fitness trainers get more pleasure from helping someone who is unfit to shape up than from fine-tuning an athlete, so never feel worried that you are being a nuisance.

6. If you have some pals at your local or workplace who want to lose a few pounds along with you, get together and encourage each other. Charity slim-ins can work but, in my experience, fellas tend to overdo it and then put the weight back on again. Don't fall into this trap. It's better to aim to take part in a fun run, in, say, a year's time when you will be fit enough to do your bit for charity.

7. Drink plenty of water – up to 3 litres daily. Men rarely drink enough water. It is essential for the health of all the cells in your body, and to keep your kidneys working properly. Aim for a pint glass of water halfway through the morning, at lunchtime and after work, and then sip steadily all through the evening. Do the 'pee' test (as recommended by superfit rugby stars): check the colour of your urine. Dark is very dodgy, lighter is better – very light means that you are drinking enough water.

8. Do your own food shopping, or go to the shops with your partner. It's important that you get your eye on the kind of foods that are available. Enjoy looking for gorgeous, fresh vegetables; the best, leanest cuts of meat and the freshest fish.

9. Go easy on salt. Many men shake salt and pepper onto their food without first tasting it. A high salt intake can cause blood pressure problems, and there is lots of 'hidden' salt in food already. Instead, use herbs, spices, lemon juice and black pepper to add oomph.

10. Don't think of your diet plan as simply a means to an end. Instead, be determined to use it as part of a major lifestyle change which will help improve your health and well-being. Oh yes, and you will have a lot more fun, as well.

DIET PLAN

DAILY ALLOWANCES

MILK
½ pint semi-skimmed milk for tea, coffee and to pour on cereals.

BOOZE
Two units of alcohol daily (that is 2 half-pints of bitter or lager, 2 glasses of wine or 2 double pub measures of spirits with low-calorie mixers only). You can save up your booze allowance for weekends if you like (a very generous 7 pints a week – not bad, eh?). Don't forget, the first pint doesn't touch the sides of your belly. Quench your thirst with a pint of water with a dash of squash or lime before you have your first beer.

FREE VEGETABLES
You can eat as much as you like from the following list of very low-calorie vegetables: asparagus, beansprouts, broccoli, Brussels sprouts, cabbage, cauliflower, celery, lettuce, mushrooms, mustard and cress, pak choi, peppers (red, green, yellow), radishes, runner beans, spinach, spring onions, tomatoes (canned and fresh), watercress, water chestnuts. Cook your vegetables lightly, or as a stir-fry (use a little water instead of oil or use very little oil and add a few tablespoons of water), and serve salads with a lemon juice and herb dressing or a tablespoon of fat-free vinaigrette dressing.

HERBS, SPICES AND SAUCES
You can also have as much as you like from the following list: freshly ground black pepper, garlic, ginger, allspice, curry powder, Chinese

five spice sauce, light soy sauce, Worcestershire sauce, oriental fish sauce, lemon and lime juice.

Every day choose one breakfast, one light meal, one main meal, two snacks and one 'diet extra' from the lists given below. (You can eat them at any time. For instance, if you work shifts, you may find it more convenient to eat your main meal at lunchtime. The diet extra is useful as a pre- or post-exercise snack.)

Important: If you have more than three stone to lose, choose THREE SNACKS daily. Eat them when you are feeling low (pull over into a lay-by if you are driving), or during the evening when you get an attack of the nibbles. (The diet allows about 1750 calories per day for men with up to 3 stone to lose; 1850 for larger chaps!)

BREAKFASTS

- Scrambled Egg with Mushrooms (see recipe, page 67), slice of wholemeal toast with scraping of low-fat spread, medium glass fruit juice
- 2 Weetabix, milk from allowance, small sliced banana
- 2 slices wholemeal toast, topped with poached egg, grilled tomatoes, watercress
- Medium bowl any cereal (including sweet cereals), milk from allowance, sliced apple, a few raisins, small glass fruit juice
- Breakfast Fruit Muffin (see recipe, page 72), 1 apple, orange or pear, small carton diet yogurt
- 1 well-grilled low fat sausage (or veggie sausage) in a small crusty roll with salad, tomatoes; 1 orange or small glass fruit juice
- 1 medium egg, boiled or poached, 2 slices of wholemeal toast with scraping of low-fat spread and 1 tsp marmalade or jam
- Fresh fruit salad: slice 1 small banana, 1 apple, 1 pear and serve topped with small carton diet yogurt and 1 tbsp muesli
- Fruit Smoothie (see recipe, page 75).

LIGHT MEALS

CANTEEN/RESTAURANT:

- Slice of melon or clear soup, 250g/10oz grilled roast chicken piece (no skin), 'free' vegetables and salad, 200g/8oz jacket potato, 2 tbsp baked beans
- Ham or chicken salad or small portion quiche with salad, 1 apple, pear or small banana
- Portion of cereal from Kellogg's Variety Pack (most canteens have them), milk from allowance, sliced banana or apple and pear, small carton diet yogurt, glass fruit juice
- 2-egg omelette with ham or mushrooms, huge 'free' salad, medium crusty rolll
- 250g/10oz grilled trout, salmon or other fish, 'free' vegetables, 2 scoops vanilla ice-cream

PACKED:

- Double-decker Sandwich (see recipe, page 99), a few grapes
- Low-fat Hummus with Pitta and Salad (see recipe, page 101), medium banana or 1 apple and 1 pear
- Any high street sandwich, flatbread or baguette of 400 calories or less, 1 piece fruit (eg. apple, pear, 2 plums)
- 1 bap or roll spread with mustard, 50g/2oz lean cold ham, beef, pork, chicken (no skin), cold cooked low-fat sausage, or Quorn Quarterpounder; small carton diet yogurt or fromage frais, 1 apple or pear
- Sandwich of 2 slices wholemeal bread spread with mustard or a little low-fat spread with lots of 'free' salad and one of these fillings: 25g/1oz grated hard cheese mixed with grated carrot and 2 tsp low-fat mayonnaise; 50g/2oz low-fat soft cheese and chopped gherkins or 2 tsp sweet pickle; Aubergine Pâté with Garlic (see recipe, page 81). Plus small carton diet yogurt and 1 apple, or 1 pack low-fat crisps, or mug of soup with crispbread for dunking

Fight Fat, Fight Fatigue Diet and Cookbook

TOASTED SNACKS

- 2 slices wholemeal toast with one of these toppings: 1 small can baked beans, spaghetti in tomato sauce or ravioli, with lots of grilled tomatoes and watercress; 1 poached egg with grilled tomatoes and salad; 1 small (125g) can tuna or salmon in brine with lemon juice, salad; 1 Quorn Quarterpounder with grilled tomatoes, salad. Plus small banana or apple and pear, or medium glass fresh fruit juice or small carton of diet yogurt with a few grapes

MAIN MEALS

- Mixed grill: medium (100g/4oz) lean lamb chop or pork tenderloin or Quorn Quarterpounder grilled, 1 rasher lean bacon or Quorn Slice, grilled, 1 low-fat sausage, grilled, 'free' vegetables and salad, 2 tbsp peas or sweetcorn, 1 apple or orange
- 200g/8oz any fish, grilled or cooked in a foil parcel in the oven with onion rings, lemon juice, tomatoes, herbs; 100g/4oz oven chips or 200g/8oz jacket potato, 'free' vegetables and salad
- Leek and Seafood Lasagne (see recipe, page 112), 'free' tomato and cucumber salad with garlic and lemon juice, fresh fruit salad (sliced apple, raspberries or strawberries, plus kiwi fruit)
- Normandy Pork (see recipe, page 109), 200g/8oz jacket potato, 'free' salad and vegetables
- Mixed Stuffed Vegetables (see recipe, page 114), 50g/2oz (cooked weight) tagliatelle or rice, 'free' salad
- Beef Casserole with Guinness (see recipe, page 118), 'free' vegetables, 3 tbsp boiled rice or 2 small boiled potatoes, baked apple with raisins, 1 tsp honey and 1 small carton low-fat fromage frais poured over
- Low-fat Moussaka (see recipe, page 108), 'free' salad topped with 50g/2oz cubed feta cheese, 1 apple or pear

- Stuffed Courgettes (see recipe, page 124), Ginger Beef Steak with Pineapple Salsa (see recipe, page 126), 'free' salad and vegetables
- Any 400 calorie rice- or pasta-based ready meal with 'free' vegetables and salad
- Large slice melon, 250g/10oz chicken piece, grilled or roasted (no skin), or Quorn Roast, 200g/7oz jacket potato or 100g/4oz oven chips, 'free' vegetables or salad

SNACKS

- Bruschetta with Parmesan (see recipe, page 82), 'free' salad
- Any Rice Cake or Crispbread Topper (see list, page 85)
- 2 jaffa cakes
- Microwaved Banana with Cinnamon (see recipe, page 87)
- Slice of toast topped with 1 tsp jam or marmalade, or 2 tsp low-fat cheese spread and tomatoes

DIET EXTRAS

- Small (150g/6oz) jacket potato
- Medium banana
- 2 fingers Kit Kat
- 1 fun-size choc bar and 1 peach, nectarine or pear

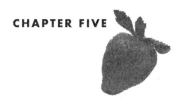

CHAPTER FIVE

TEEN EATING PLAN

Healthy menus to help you keep fit and trim

A re you aged between 13 and 19 – and are you anxious to look and feel great? What a daft question! Of course, everyone who is young wants to be trim and fit. You long to look trendy – with slinky hips, a flat tum and sensational legs – just like your favourite movie or pop star. If you feel lumpy and dumpy, it's useless parents and friends saying 'you look fine'. There is nothing 'fine' about being the largest person in the class, or being too big to wear the latest, figure-hugging clothes.

While it's a lousy idea for a youngster to follow a crazy diet plan (and there are plenty of those around), it makes sense to eat healthily, without getting 'hung up' about food. Of course, it is also important to take plenty of exercise – though you certainly don't need to become a fitness addict.

So how do you find a 'happy' weight and fitness level for yourself? The best way is to follow my tips and easy eating plan, and to get a copy of the companion book in this series, *Firm Up All Over,* by GMTV fitness expert Nicki Waterman, which will help you find an exercise regime to suit you.

Here are ten facts that you should know before you start:

1. Your shape is governed by genetic factors. If your mum and dad are both tall with a large frame, there is no way you are going to look like pint-size popster Kylie Minogue. Similarly, if your parents are small and dumpy, there is a strong possibility that you will be small and well covered too – so forget aiming for the leggy, Kate Moss silhouette. What you should do is aim to be the best 'you' that you can be.

2. You are very special, talented and gorgeous. Who says so? YOU do. When we are born, we have no hang-ups about our bodies, looks or abilities – we have to learn them. If you feel less than happy about yourself, replace those negative thoughts with positive ones. Make a list of all your good points. I bet there are loads.

3. Food is fun, vital for good looks and health, and should be enjoyed. Many youngsters grow up in an atmosphere where food is associated with guilt. They are told that certain things are 'naughty' (perhaps your

---

mum is on a diet and keeps on moaning about chocolate cravings, or worrying about her passion for pizza?) and, somehow, that idea takes hold. Remember: all food is OK – what's important is to get the balance right. You need carbs to fuel your muscles, and protein for growth. Some fat is also essential to a healthy diet as it provides vitamins A, D and E and essential fatty acids which the body cannot manufacture. However, the type of fat consumed is important. Saturated fat (found mainly in animal products) has been associated with an increased risk of coronary heart disease and cancer, so should be eaten in moderation. Unsaturated fat (found in oily fish, soya beans, walnuts, wheatgerm) is as high in calories as saturated but has health benefits as well.

Some things like fruit, fresh vegetables, fish, lean meat and lower fat dairy foods are good to eat often because they help you build a healthy body, and do lots for your looks. Others – like fatty takeaways, crisps and chocs – are less healthy and should be eaten less often. But, no foods are taboo. Even sugar, although much-maligned, is OK in moderation. So the occasional tube of wine gums or dollop of jam on your bread is fine.

45

4. You are still growing and developing. Your body is changing all the time, so give it a good chance to become strong and beautiful by eating well.

5. You don't have to believe everything you read and see on telly – especially where slimming and nutrition are concerned. Recently we have been exposed to a crop of scary TV programmes, crack-pot articles about 'miracle' pills, and magazines devoted to so-called 'star' slimming and fitness secrets. Treat all such rubbish with the deepest suspicion. If in doubt, contact me at my email address for advice, and the truth (see page 150).

6. Eating breakfast will improve your figure and make you brainier. Oh yes it will! Numerous studies have shown that people who eat a sensible,

balanced breakfast (such as cereal, toast, fruit juice) are more likely to be slim than people who skip breakfast. What's more, it is known that eating breakfast helps you to concentrate, perform better and feel less tired – all day long.

7. Cooking is fun. If you learn to prepare delicious, healthy meals you will get in shape. You will also be very popular with your family and friends, especially if you are at college and living on a budget. Most important, you will be in control of what you put into your mouth. So if you haven't yet been very keen on cooking, now is the time to try. Many of the recipes in this book are an absolute doddle to prepare. Have a go.

8. Drinking lots of water will improve your skin and beef up your energy levels. Fizzy drinks are loaded with sugar and chemicals, and should only be drunk occasionally. When you go out, try sipping mineral water or non-fizzy water with orange juice – you could start a trend. Alcohol is very fattening and it makes people lose control so they eat too much of the wrong things and behave stupidly. Just think about some of the older people you know. Enough said.

9. You will work harder and study more effectively if you allow time for exercise and eating properly. Even when important exams are looming, allow some time for a daily walk, swim or cycle ride. Keep fruit on your desk for nibbling, water to drink, and have a milky 'nightcap' to help you sleep. Always keep one or two of the snacks listed at the end of the section in your workbag so you are not at the mercy of the school tuckshop or college snack bar.

10. Bullies are sad, not bad. If you are teased about your shape, feel sorry for the person who is making the jibe. After all, you are well on the way

to improving your looks while they are stuck with an appalling personality defect! If you are always first to crack a joke about yourself (to get it in before anyone else does), stop being such a dummy. Go back and read number two.

YOUR HEALTHY NUTRITION PROGRAMME

This plan can be followed by teenage girls or boys who are trying to regulate their body weight and become leaner. The calorie allowance is 1800 daily, with extra calories if you are playing sport regularly. (I advise you to get a copy of Nicki Waterman's book in this series, *Firm Up All Over*. It includes plenty of ideas on how to have fun exercising.)

The diet is high in carbohydrate (about 250g/10oz daily) because this is vital to fuel your muscles for exercise, and to fill you up. A great deal of work on this subject has been carried out by Professor Anne de Looy of Queen Margaret University College, Edinburgh. Professor de Looy has found that increasing the amount of carbs (bread, pasta, potatoes, even sweet foods like jam) in the diet helps you stop overeating the fattier foods like chips and burgers. Our Fight Fat, Fight Fatigue theory is that by eating well and having regular, carb-rich snacks you will feel livelier and be more inclined to exercise.

Daily Allowances and Guidelines

MILK
Allow ¾ pint semi-skimmed milk for cereals and tea or coffee (try to limit cups to three daily).

FREE VEGETABLES

You can eat as much as you like from the following list of very low-calorie vegetables: Asparagus, beansprouts, broccoli, Brussels sprouts, cabbage, cauliflower, celery, lettuce, mushrooms, mustard and cress, pak choi, peppers (red, green, yellow), radishes, runner beans, spinach, spring onions, tomatoes (canned and fresh), watercress, water chestnuts.

If you 'hate' vegetables, give them another chance. Salads can be very tasty if you choose a wide variety of ingredients instead of limp lettuce and squashed tomatoes; and green vegetables such as cabbage and leeks are delicious lightly cooked with herbs, garlic, lemon juice and other vegetables such as tomatoes and onions.

WATER

Drink at least 3 litres of water daily. If you are taking regular exercise or playing sport, you should drink plenty of water before and after your workout or match. If you want to be scientific about it, we need a basic level of about 40ml/1½ fl oz of water for every kilo of body weight. So, if you weigh, say 60kg/132lb, you need at least 2½ litres/4½ pints of water. This obviously increases during hot weather. Try to swap at least some of your daily fizzy drinks for water – you'll be amazed at how much more energetic you feel.

BREAD

You can have any kind of bread on this diet, so don't feel worried if you prefer the sliced white kind to wholemeal – it's not as good but it's still OK. Bread is not a 'baddie' by the way – it's an essential source of carbs and calcium to help build healthy bones.

VEGETARIAN CHOICES

There are plenty of items for veggies. Make sure you vary your diet, and have adequate iron (dark green leafy vegetables) and vitamin B (wholegrain cereals, bread, pasta). Don't be tempted to fill up with biscuits and chocs when your mates have a burger – most high street restaurants now have veggie options.

Choose one breakfast, one lunch, one supper, three snacks and, if you are playing sports, one 'diet extra' from the lists below. Follow the plan for a couple of weeks, while stepping up the amount of exercise you take – whether it is sports at school or college, dancing, walking or swimming. At the end of the two weeks you will feel fitter and healthier. You can then use this plan as the basis for your own eating programme, ringing the changes with recipes chosen from the Recipe section (pages 63–148), or your own choice of meals. Don't forget that NO food is taboo – just use your common sense and make sure the majority of your diet is made up of healthy food.

49

BREAKFASTS

- 2 Weetabix, milk from allowance, sliced apple, a few raisins or dried apricots; 1 slice toast with 1 tsp jam or marmalade
- 2 slices toast topped with small can (150g/6oz) baked beans, grilled tomatoes, watercress, mushrooms poached in water; small glass fruit juice
- BLT sandwich: spread 2 slices bread with mild mustard and fill with 1 well-grilled rasher lean back bacon, lettuce, tomato, cucumber and watercress. Munch with small glass fruit juice or, if you are eating it on the bus, a couple of satsumas
- Apple and Lime Crunchie (see recipe, page 68), small glass fruit juice
- 1 carton cereal from a Kellogg's Variety Pack, milk from allowance, medium sliced banana or sliced apple and pear, medium glass fruit juice

- Apple and Blackberry Pancakes (see recipe, page 76), small carton diet yogurt
- Medium egg (boiled or poached), grilled tomatoes, watercress, 2 slices toast, 1 tsp jam or marmalade

LUNCHES

- Bean and Vegetable Soup (see recipe, page 93), crusty roll, 1 apple or pear
- Low-fat Hummus (see recipe, page 101) with pitta bread and salad, 1 medium banana

PACKED:

- Sandwich of 2 slices bread or small split baguette roll with one of the following fillings and accompaniments, plus plenty of 'free' salad: 50g/2oz lean cold meat (no skin or fat) or Quorn Deli Slices, or two cold cooked low-fat or veggie sausages, plus 1 medium banana or apple and pear; 50g/2oz low-fat cheese spread, meat or fish paste or sandwich spread, small carton fruit juice, 1 satsuma

HIGH STREET/CANTEEN/RESTAURANT:

- Any 350-calorie sandwich, roll, flatbread or pitta (eg. Boots Shapers), or portion of sushi, 1 packet low-fat crisps, 1 apple, orange, pear or small carton fruit drink
- 1 medium beefburger or vegeburger (or equivalent), grilled, bun, salad, 2 tsp relish or tomato sauce, huge 'free' salad, 1 medium banana
- 2 slices toast topped with poached egg and baked beans, medium glass fruit juice, 1 apple or 2 satsumas or medium portion strawberries or raspberries

- Medium (220g/8oz) jacket potato with baked bean, coleslaw or tuna filling, huge portion of salad, 1 apple, pear or small banana
- 50g/2oz any cold, lean meat, or 150g/6oz any grilled fish without batter, or medium portion quiche, huge portion 'free' salad, medium jacket potato, 1 apple, pear or portion fresh fruit salad or strawberries

SUPPERS

- Chicken Maryland (see recipe, page 106), 'free' salad and vegetables
- Polynesian Beef Stir-fry (see recipe, page 107), 50g/2oz (cooked weight) noodles or rice, 'free' vegetables, 2 scoops vanilla ice-cream and 2 wafers with sliced peach or strawberries on top
- Cod steak in wholemeal crumb or mushroom or parsley sauce (Birds Eye or similar brand), 'free' vegetables, 2 medium boiled potatoes, fruit-flavoured jelly
- Large slice melon, 50g/2oz any lean roast meat or Quorn Roast, 'free' vegetables, medium roast potato or 2 medium boiled potatoes, low-fat fromage frais or small carton low-fat yogurt
- 50g/2oz (cooked weight) any pasta with sauce made from ½ jar low-fat Dolmio cook-in tomato sauce mixed with 50g/2oz lean beef mince or 75g/3oz Quorn pieces, garlic, herbs, huge 'free' salad, 1 apple or pear
- Leek and Seafood Lasagne (see recipe, page 112), huge 'free' salad, low-fat fromage frais or fruit yogurt with sliced, fresh peach or medium portion strawberries or raspberries
- Any 400-calorie pasta- or rice-based ready meal, 'free' vegetables or salad, sliced peach, mango or nectarine with 1 scoop vanilla ice-cream

SNACKS (Choose three – eat at any time, particularly after sports, washed down with plenty of water)

- Any Rice Cake or Crispbread Topper (see list, page 85)
- 1 medium banana or 1 apple and 1 orange or pear
- Slice of bread topped with 1 tsp jam or Marmite with tomatoes and watercress
- 2 jaffa cakes
- Small packet of wine gums, jelly babies or fun-size choc bar

DIET EXTRAS (Choose one – eat about 1½ hrs before exercising)

- 1 medium bowl cereal chosen from Kellogg's Variety Pack with milk from allowance
- Microwaved Banana with Cinnamon (see recipe, page 87), small glass fruit juice
- Bruschetta with Parmesan (see recipe, page 82), 1 apple

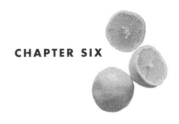

CHAPTER SIX

HOW TO MAINTAIN YOUR WEIGHT LOSS

All you need to know about staying slim forever

The most often quoted comment about slimming is 'anyone can shed weight ... the difficult bit is keeping it off'. How true. However, while various sets of depressing statistics show that many people do regain some, or indeed all, of the weight they have shed, it is also true that those who make permanent changes to their lifestyle and combine a sensible diet with exercise DO stay in shape.

The Fight Fat, Fight Fatigue programme helps you to improve your energy levels as well as lose weight, and encourages you to take regular exercise, so it is the best possible plan to follow.

If you have now reached your 'happy weight' and feel fitter and more energetic than you have ever felt in your life, there are many things you can do to ensure that you stay on top form. Here's my ten-point guide:

1. **Recognize old patterns and change them** Be aware that the human brain is the world's most sophisticated computer and can store minute details of our lives and experiences – and dig them out at the most inappropriate times. This means that if you have been a binge-eater, or had a passion for chocs, or went through a period of never eating breakfast, it is quite possible that you could drift back into those habits. Binges, for instance, are often triggered by an emotional upset. If this does happen, don't feel guilty – and don't for goodness sake say 'oh well I've blown it now anyway' – just resolve to go back to your healthy lifestyle as quickly as possible. Remember that however upsetting things are, you will be able to deal with them more effectively if you stay fit.

2. **Watch out for creeping weight gain** Set yourself a 2.5kg/5lb 'ceiling' of weight gain and once that has been passed, use the Quick Weight-loss plan in Chapter 2 – to get yourself back down to your best weight. Don't let the pounds creep on and on. I am not in favour of the 'stop-start' attitude to eating which means losing a load of weight for Christmas, eating like crazy over the holiday, then resolving to lose those excess pounds in January. Moderation is the key to successful weight maintenance. Even on holiday, try to enjoy the freshest, most delicious foods, but don't feel you have to eat all day. Boozing is fun occasionally, but

not every weekend. Why waste precious free time feeling under the weather?

3. **Keep it up** Keep on exercising, every single day. Studies have shown that people who exercise earlier in the day are most likely to stick with it. So, go for that morning run or early morning swim. In cold weather, wrap up warmly and reward yourself with a hot toddy when you come back. In summer, when there are many distractions, get up half an hour earlier to fit your exercise into your schedule.

4. **Have a re-fit** Get rid of all your 'fat' clothes. Why keep your old baggy leggings, or 40in waist trousers at the back of the wardrobe? Are you willing yourself to fail? Be bold and chuck out the unflattering outfits you hated to wear while you were carrying those excess pounds. You simply don't need them any more.

55

5. **Enjoy yourself** Enjoy all the pluses of being slimmer. Book up for all those trips you avoided because you felt too self-conscious to use public transport, or too embarrassed to squeeze your body into a plane or train seat. Go swimming, socialize – use your new energy to pack your life with interesting hobbies and new projects. Activity keeps you young and slim.

6. **Resist the pressure** Don't be influenced by other people. I've talked to many slimmers who have drifted back into their bad old eating habits because of pressure from partners or friends. Once they 'finished' dieting, they faced thoughtless comments like: 'great, now we can have some decent grub around here for a change' or 'good, let's go down to the pub and I can buy you a few real drinks.' You are the one who has made the changes, and you

are the one who has most to lose by failing, so stick to your guns. There is no need to have rows, just be firm. Remember that many people feel threatened when their loved ones become slimmer and fitter. Be loving and caring, but don't be rail-roaded into fattening up.

7. **Don't become a diet bore** Enjoy cooking low-fat dishes, but don't make a meal of it! Your mates will soon get fed up if you invite them over for a 'low-fat' supper and then bore them silly with tales of your own success. Use the delicious dinner party menus on pages 121–35, but don't even mention that the dishes are low in fat. They'll never guess, anyway.

8. **Look after your health** Have regular health and fitness check-ups. By losing weight and shaping up you have extended your life expectancy and improved your day-to-day quality of living. Keep on top of any creaks, aches and hidden problems with regular checks. Never ignore symptoms which are odd, or worrying, such as loss of appetite, unusual levels of tiredness, or frequent passing of urine.

9. **Treat yourself – mind and body** Every day, save an hour for yourself. Read, listen to music, or have a hair-do, go to an exhibition or just window-shop for a new outfit. Even if you are pressured at work, or have a demanding family, you need to 'feed' your mind and ego, as well as your body. A well-nourished brain is very useful if you are trying to maintain a well-nourished body.

10. **Keep reading this book** Make sure it is kept on the kitchen shelf, so you can use it every day to help you cook up the delicious recipes. Re-read these tips while you are waiting for the toast to pop up or the kettle to boil.

Fight Fat, Fight Fatigue Diet and Cookbook

DIET PLAN

This plan is great for anyone wanting to maintain their present weight. It shows you how to adjust your calorie intake to a suitable level for weight maintenance. It contains 1700 calories, which is too low if you are exercising regularly and are at target.

Weigh in on a Monday, follow the diet for two weeks, then weigh yourself again. If your weight is still falling, raise your calorie intake using one of the 100 calorie diet boosters listed on page 61. Continue for another week, and add another diet booster, and so on, until your weight stays the same.

As everyone is different, this can only be a general guide. The level of exercise you do is very important as well. For instance, if your activity consists of a great deal of aerobic training, you could continue to shed weight unless you increase your calorie intake even more. If you have become very active since following our diet and exercise programme (and I hope you have), then get some advice from your own personal trainer or resident gym nutritionist.

Daily Allowances and Guidelines

MILK
Allow yourself ½ pint of semi-skimmed milk for cereals, tea and coffee (keep cuppas to 3 daily).

DRINKS
1 glass dry wine or ½ pint beer or lager daily (you can have it on two 'nights out' if you prefer). Drink 6–8 glasses of water as well (low-calorie soft drinks should be kept to a minimum).

FREE VEGETABLES

You can eat as much as you like from the following list of very low-calorie vegetables: Asparagus, beansprouts, broccoli, Brussels sprouts, cabbage, cauliflower, celery, lettuce, mushrooms, mustard and cress, pak choi, peppers (red, green, yellow), radishes, runner beans, spinach, spring onions, tomatoes (canned and fresh), watercress, water chestnuts.

HERBS, SPICES AND SAUCES

You can also have as much as you like from the following list: freshly ground black pepper, garlic, ginger, allspice, curry powder, Chinese five spice sauce, light soy sauce, Worcestershire sauce, oriental fish sauce, lemon and lime juice.

Now choose one breakfast, one lunch, one supper and two snacks daily. You may swap the lunches and suppers if you wish (for instance if you have a Sunday lunch or are a shift worker). Remember to add extra Diet Boosters if you continue to lose weight.

BREAKFAST

- Well-grilled rasher back bacon, poached egg, 1 slice toast, grilled tomatoes, mushrooms cooked in stock, small glass fruit juice
- Apple and Lime Crunchie (see recipe, page 68), 1 slice toast with 1 tsp jam or marmalade, small glass fruit juice
- Smoked Cod Kedgeree (see recipe, page 70), grilled tomatoes, watercress, 2 crispbreads
- Honey Baked Apple (see recipe, page 71), 1 slice toast with 1 tsp honey or jam, small banana, small glass fruit juice
- Egg and Bacon Soufflé Omelette (see recipe, page 73), grilled tomatoes, watercress, medium glass fruit juice

- Fruit Smoothie (see recipe, page 75), small sweet biscuit for dunking
- 50g/2oz serving any cereal such as Special K with Red Berries or Fruit 'n' Fibre, muesli, milk from allowance, medium sliced banana
- 2 slices toast topped with 1 small can (150g/6oz) baked beans mixed with 1 tbsp sweetcorn, watercress, grilled tomatoes; small glass fruit juice
- Scrambled Egg with Mushrooms (see recipe, page 67), 50g/2oz smoked salmon, 1 slice toast, small glass fruit juice

LUNCHES

PACKED:

- Chicken and Ham Pâté with Oriental Salad (see recipe, page 92), 1 apple, pear or orange
- Curried Chicken Breasts with Spicy Carrot Dip (see recipe, page 94), small bunch grapes or 2 satsumas
- Stuffed Peppers with Creamy Coleslaw (see recipe, page 96), small crusty roll, medium portion strawberries or raspberries
- Double-decker Sandwich (see recipe, page 99), a few grapes
- 50g/2oz any cold, cooked lean meat or Quorn Deli Slices, huge salad from 'free' list, one portion Fruity Bread Pudding (see recipe, page 103).
- 2 slices bread or medium crusty roll or pitta bread with one of these fillings and accompaniments:100g/4oz can tuna or salmon in brine, 'free' salad sprinkled with lemon juice, small banana; small carton (150g/6oz) cottage cheese (plain or with pineapple or chives), 'free' salad, 1 apple, 1 pear; cold cooked low-fat sausage or veggie sausage, 1 dsp sweet pickle or relish, 'free' salad, 1 kiwi fruit or 2 plums

HIGH STREET/CANTEEN/RESTAURANT:

- Any 350-calorie sandwich, flatbread, pitta bread or sushi (eg. Boots Shapers), plus 1 apple, pear, orange or kiwi fruit and a large portion 'free' salad

How to Maintain Your Weight Loss

- Slice of melon, 50g/2oz any cold, cooked lean meat, medium (220g/8oz) jacket potato, 'free' salad, small carton low-fat fruit yogurt
- Medium (220g/8oz) jacket potato with baked bean, tuna or coleslaw topping, 'free' salad, apple, orange, or small banana
- Italian restaurant meal of pasta with clams or tomato sauce, huge mixed salad, small crusty roll
- Burger bar meal of hamburger with bun (no onions), salad, medium glass fruit juice, 1 apple

SUPPERS

- Normandy Pork (see recipe, page 109), 'free' vegetables and salad, 2 medium boiled potatoes, fresh fruit salad made with raspberries, sliced apple and sliced mango
- Pears Roquefort (see recipe, page 125), 50g/2oz cold, lean meat, canned fish (pilchards, salmon etc.), or Quorn Deli slices, huge salad from 'free' list, crusty roll, small carton low-fat yogurt
- Slice of melon, Leek and Seafood Lasagne (see recipe, page 112), huge mixed salad from 'free' list, Honey-Baked Apple (see recipe, page 71)
- 50g/2oz any lean, roast meat or Quorn Roast, 2 medium roast potatoes, thin gravy, 'free' vegetables, 125g/4oz low-fat fromage frais or Chocolate Mousse with Rum (see recipe, page 133)
- Slimmers' soup (any flavour), crusty roll, Plaice with Mustard Sauce (see recipe, page 115), 'free' vegetables, 75g/3oz mashed potato (using milk from allowance), 1 apple or pear
- Beef Casserole with Guinness (see recipe, page 118), 'free' vegetables, 75g/3oz mashed potato (using milk from allowance), small carton low-fat fruit yogurt poured over sliced mango or peach
- 200g/8oz any oily fish (trout, mackerel, salmon) grilled with lemon juice and herbs, 'free' salad and vegetables, 50g/2oz (cooked weight) pasta or rice or 100g/4oz oven chips, 125g/4oz low-fat fromage frais

Fight Fat, Fight Fatigue Diet and Cookbook

- 200g/8oz any shellfish (crab, lobster, prawns) served cooked and cold with 2 tbsp low-fat mayonnaise for dunking, 'free' salad with lots of lemon juice, 1 crusty roll, fresh fruit salad made with sliced apple, small sliced banana, raspberries or strawberries

SNACKS

- 1 packet low-fat crisps
- 2 jaffa cakes
- 1 small banana
- Any Rice Cake, Crispbread or Meringue Nest Topper (see recipes, pages 85 and 86)
- 1 apple and 2 plums
- 1 kiwi fruit and 1 pear
- 1 fun-size choc bar
- 2 fingers Kit Kat

61

100-CALORIE DIET BOOSTERS

- 1 crusty roll with 'free' salad
- 2 small boiled potatoes
- 50g/2oz (cooked weight) pasta or rice
- Boiled or poached egg
- 1 rasher well-grilled lean back bacon
- 1 low-fat sausage
- 1 mug hot chocolate or other nightcap (made with milk from allowance) and 1 small biscuit
- 25g/1oz serving breakfast cereal
- Kelloggs Special K bar

THE RECIPES

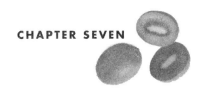

CHAPTER SEVEN

BRILLIANT BREAKFASTS

A delicious, nutritious start to your day

Many thousands of words have been written about the importance of breakfast. There's even a national 'breakfast week' every year, promoting the benefits of eating a sensible, balanced meal first thing in the morning. Even so, at least 25 per cent of the population go to work, college or school with empty tummies. That's a big shame. Quite apart from the nutritional importance of the meal, eating breakfast has a very beneficial effect for anyone trying to lose weight. It's been proved in many pieces of research that people who eat breakfast are more alert and less likely to snack on junk foods than those who go without.

So, if you want to feel lively, and shed that excess weight as well, make time for breakfast. You don't have to eat the same, boring things every day, either. Below are ten quickie recipes which are delicious and easy to prepare. Try them as part of your diet plan. They are also suitable for all members of the family. (Add extra toast, fruit and juice for growing teenagers, and men!)

All recipes serve four (apart from Breakfast Fruit Muffins).

SCRAMBLED EGG WITH MUSHROOMS

4 medium eggs
Seasoning to taste
2 x 156g/6oz cans button mushrooms, drained
Watercress for garnish

Beat the eggs in a bowl, and season lightly. Heat the mushrooms in a pan. Cook the eggs in the microwave oven on High for 30 seconds, then stir, and repeat. Mix the mushrooms and eggs, garnish with watercress and serve.

CALORIES PER SERVING: 150   FAT: 6.6G

Nutrition notes: *Eggs are a good source of protein and iron, while the mushrooms add some fibre and small amounts of vitamin B. To aid absorption of the iron, you could add a small glass of orange juice to this meal.*

67

APPLE AND LIME CRUNCHIE

This is a perfect breakfast dish because it contains many nutrients.

450g/1lb cooking apples, peeled, cored and sliced
2 tbsp freshly squeezed lime juice
2 tbsp water
Artificial sweetener to taste
150g/5oz natural, unsweetened yogurt
4 tbsp muesli, lightly toasted
4 tbsp lime curd or lime marmalade
4 thin slices lime for garnish

Put the apple slices into a pan with the lime juice and water. Cover and simmer gently until the apples are soft and pulpy. Add artificial sweetener to taste. Chill overnight. Before breakfast, fold the yogurt into the apple mixture. Put half the mixture into 4 tall glasses, sprinkle the toasted muesli over the top, add a spoonful of lime curd or marmalade, and top with the remaining apple mixture. Decorate each glass with a twisted lime slice and serve immediately. (This recipe works well with orange marmalade or lemon curd instead of lime, plus a twist of orange or slice of kiwi fruit.)

CALORIES PER SERVING: 200   FAT: 1G

Nutrition notes: *Apples are a good source of vitamin C, and provide fibre and carbohydrate. The lime juice also contains vitamin C, and the muesli has B vitamins, fibre and carbohydrate. The natural yogurt provides protein and calcium. Have a nice day!*

HAREM BREAKFAST

2 tbsp blanched almonds, split
1 bunch watercress, coarse stems removed, washed and roughly chopped
2 large oranges, peeled and thinly sliced
100g/4oz cottage cheese
50g/2oz fresh or dried dates, roughly chopped

Grill the almonds on a baking sheet, shaking to turn them, so they brown evenly on all sides. Arrange the prepared watercress and orange slices around the inside of four sundae glasses. Top with the cottage cheese, and arrange the dates and toasted almonds on top.

CALORIES PER SERVING: 115   FAT: 3G

Nutrition notes: *Almonds contain protein and are rich in vitamins and minerals including potassium, calcium and magnesium. Watercress contains iron, oranges have vitamin C, and cottage cheese is a good source of protein and calcium. Dates are also rich in magnesium and calcium and they contain copper, which helps strengthen the nervous system.*

SMOKED COD KEDGEREE

This breakfast dish was traditionally served as a colonial 'filler', as it provided the good start needed by men going off on a long day's trek.

225g/8oz brown rice
Salt
1 small onion, finely chopped
1 tsp olive oil
2 tbsp natural, unsweetened yogurt
175g/6oz smoked cod, cooked and flaked
1 hard-boiled egg, roughly chopped
2 tbsp chopped fresh flat-leaf parsley
Freshly ground black pepper
Paprika to garnish

Cook the brown rice in boiling, salted water for about 20 minutes until just tender. Drain thoroughly. Fry the onion gently in the olive oil until soft, 3–4 minutes. Add the drained, cooked rice, and stir over the heat for a further 3–4 minutes. Add the yogurt, fish, chopped egg, chopped parsley and pepper to taste. Stir over the heat until all ingredients are heated through. Garnish with paprika before serving.

CALORIES PER SERVING: 370   FAT: 2.2G

Nutrition notes: *Brown rice is a good source of vitamin B plus fibre, and the smoked cod and egg provide protein and iron. Parsley is surprisingly rich in iron, folate and betacarotene. In large quantities it can have a natural diuretic (water chasing) effect, too.*

HONEY-BAKED APPLES

These are a very comforting breakfast treat.

4 large Bramley or other cooking apples
1 tbsp clear honey
Grated rind and juice of 1 lemon
1 tbsp low-fat spread
4 tbsp low-fat natural or Greek yogurt

Preheat the oven to 180°C/350°F/Gas Mark 4. Remove the cores from the apples, taking care not to go right through the apples. Using a sharp knife, cut vertical lines through the apple skin at intervals. Stand in an ovenproof dish. Mix together the honey, lemon rind and low-fat spread. Spoon into the apples, and cover the dish with foil. Bake for 40–45 minutes or until the apples are tender. Serve hot or cold with 1 tbsp yogurt per person.

CALORIES PER SERVING: 85   FAT: 2G

Nutrition notes: *The apples contain vitamin C and carbohydrates, and the lemon juice is rich in vitamin C. Honey is carb-rich, and lubricates the throat.*

BREAKFAST FRUIT MUFFINS

These are a good choice for a quick breakfast food, and excellent for children.

225g/8oz self-raising wholemeal flour
2 tsp baking powder
2 tbsp light muscovado sugar
25g/1oz dried apricots or figs, finely chopped
1 medium banana, mashed with 1 tsp orange juice
1 tsp finely grated orange rind
300ml/10fl oz skimmed milk
1 medium egg, beaten
3 tbsp corn oil
2 tbsp porridge oats

Preheat the oven to 200°C/400°F/Gas Mark 6. Place 10 paper muffin cases in a deep tin. Sift the flour and baking powder into a bowl, stir in the sugar and dried fruit. Make a well in the centre and add the banana, orange rind, milk, beaten egg and oil. Mix to form a thick batter and divide evenly among the paper cases. Sprinkle with porridge oats and bake for 25–30 minutes, until well risen and firm to the touch. Allow to cool slightly before serving with fresh fruit or juice.

MAKES: 10   CALORIES PER MUFFIN: 185   FAT: 1.7G

Nutrition notes: *Wholemeal flour is a good source of B vitamins, and dried fruit contains potassium and magnesium. Banana provides potassium and easily digestible carbohydrate, and the orange juice supplies vitamin C. The porridge oats help lower cholesterol.*

EGG AND BACON SOUFFLÉ OMELETTE

This would be a filling and delicious choice for a family Sunday brunch. Serve with orange juice and wholemeal toast.

2 rashers lean back bacon
175g/6oz cherry tomatoes, halved
225g/8oz mushrooms, sliced
4 tbsp vegetable stock
Freshly ground black pepper
4 medium eggs, separated
4 medium egg whites
4 tsp olive oil
Small salad leaves (eg. rocket) and parsley to serve

Grill the bacon until crisp. Meanwhile, place the tomatoes and mushrooms in a pan and add the stock. Season with pepper and simmer for 5–6 minutes until tender. Drain.

Whisk the egg yolks with 4 tablespoons of water until frothy. In another bowl, beat the 8 egg whites until stiff. Fold the yolk mixture into the egg whites carefully. Brush a small omelette pan with 1 teaspoon of the olive oil, heat and pour in a quarter of the egg mixture. Cook for 4–5 minutes, then pop the pan under the grill for a couple of minutes to finish cooking. Transfer to a warm plate, fill with chopped bacon and the tomato and mushroom mixture, fold, and garnish with salad leaves and parsley. Repeat procedure for the remaining omelettes.

CALORIES PER SERVING: 240   FAT: 11G

Nutrition notes: *Eggs and bacon provide iron and protein. Tomatoes contain vitamin C, and mushrooms are high in potassium with good amounts of vitamin E and selenium, and some B vitamins.*

Brilliant Breakfasts

CHEESY TOMATOES WITH SODA BREAD

This is a quick, easy breakfast that's healthy too.

2 tsp olive oil
6 large ripe tomatoes, thickly sliced
4 thick slices soda bread
125g/4oz carton cottage cheese
Balsamic vinegar or Worcestershire sauce for drizzling

Brush a griddle pan with the olive oil, and heat. Add the tomato slices and cook for about 4 minutes, turning once, until softened and slightly blackened. Meanwhile, lightly toast the bread. Place the tomatoes on top of the toast, add a tablespoon of cottage cheese, then drizzle each portion with balsamic vinegar or Worcestershire sauce.

CALORIES PER SERVING: 150   FAT: 3.7G

Nutrition notes: *The tomatoes contain vitamins C and E, and the soda bread is carb-rich. The cottage cheese provides calcium and protein.*

FRUIT SMOOTHIE

A refreshing breakfast-in-a-hurry.

4 medium bananas, quartered
450g/1lb strawberries or raspberries
4 tbsp porridge oats
2 x 500g/17oz cartons natural, unsweetened yogurt
Ground cinnamon or nutmeg and fresh mint to garnish

Place all ingredients (except the garnish) in a food processor or blender and blend until creamy. Pour into four tall glasses, garnish and serve.

CALORIES PER SERVING: 320   FAT: 4G

Nutrition notes: *This is the ultimate high-energy drink, with plenty of carbohydrate, vitamin C, calcium and protein. Ring the changes by using other seasonal fruit such as peaches or nectarines, and vegetables such as carrot or beetroot. You can also swap the yogurt for orange or cranberry juice, which will reduce the calorie and fat content.*

APPLE AND BLACKBERRY PANCAKES

125g/4oz wholemeal flour
300ml/10fl oz skimmed milk
1 egg, beaten
1 tsp sunflower oil
Sunflower spray oil
125g/4oz low-fat natural yogurt
Sesame seeds for sprinkling

FILLING:
450g/1lb Bramley or other cooking apples
225g/8oz blackberries
3 tbsp water
2 tbsp sugar

Put the flour into a bowl, make a well in the centre and pour in a little of the milk, the egg and the teaspoon of oil. Whisk the flour into the liquid, and gradually whisk in the rest of the milk, keeping the mixture smooth. Let the mixture rest while you prepare the filling. Quarter, peel, core and slice the apples. Place the slices in a pan with the blackberries and water. Cook gently for 10–15 minutes and add the sugar to sweeten.

Spray a non-stick pan evenly with oil, let it get hot, and pour in a quarter of the pancake mixture. Cook for about 1 minute, flip over and cook the other side. Make four pancakes, and fill with the fruit mixture. Serve topped with yogurt and sesame seeds.

CALORIES PER SERVING: 150   FAT: 3G

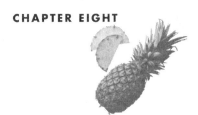

CHAPTER EIGHT

SCRUMMY SNACKS AND NIBBLES

Love at first bite!

M̶ost diets discourage slimmers from eating between meals. Fight Fat, Fight Fatigue is one plan where eating snacks is positively encouraged. There are several reasons for this.

Firstly, part of the whole 'package', the process of getting into shape and staying in shape, is to combine regular exercise with healthy eating. Time and again, slimmers fail to keep their weight off because they don't exercise. Exercise doesn't just burn off calories: it gives a feeling of well-being, decreases appetite (yes, really) and makes you feel good about yourself. However, when you exercise you need 'fuel', and that means a regular intake of nutrients, particularly carbohydrate (in fruit, vegetables, pasta, bread), which provides the instant energy you need when you work out in the gym, go swimming or cycling etc. Think of your muscles as elastic bands which need to be stretched before they can 'ping' into action: without carbohydrate to provide glycogen to fuel them, your poor muscles are like old knicker elastic – limp and saggy.

So that's why we recommend eating at least two snack-meals daily (more if you are a bloke, a teenager or on our maintenance programme, see pages 34 and 61).

Simple snacks are easy to prepare – a banana and a couple of glasses of water, for instance, is brilliant for rehydrating your body and providing carbohydrate and potassium – and a selection of quickie ideas is given in each diet plan. But sometimes you might like to take a little bit more trouble and make something extra special. The ideas on the next few pages are fun and attractive enough to be given to friends as hors d'oeuvres or as part of a party buffet. They are all 100 calories or less per portion, and very low in fat.

CRUDITÉS WITH SALSA AND CREAMY DIPS

2 red and 2 yellow peppers, seeded and sliced lengthways
225g/8oz fresh baby corn cobs, blanched
1 chicory head, trimmed and leaves separated
Small bunch radishes, trimmed
175g/6oz cherry tomatoes
6 medium carrots, cut into sticks
2 hard-boiled eggs, peeled

SALSA DIP:
400g/14oz can chopped tomatoes with herbs and garlic
Pinch chilli powder
Chopped spring onion

CREAMY DIP:
125g/4oz low-fat fromage frais
2 tbsp any low-fat salad dressing

Arrange the prepared vegetables on a serving plate together with the eggs, cut into quarters. Mix the ingredients for the dressings and serve separately for dipping.

Serves: 4

CALORIES PER PORTION – CRUDITÉS: 65   SALSA DIP: 17   CREAMY DIP: 33
FAT PER PORTION – CRUDITÉS: NEG   SALSA DIP: 0G   CREAMY DIP:0.46G

Nutrition notes: *One red pepper contains as much vitamin C as three oranges, sweetcorn contains betacarotene, eggs are protein-rich and the yolks contain iron as well. The fromage frais contains calcium for healthy bones, and even the chilli powder is good news – it helps protect the immune system.*

FENNEL AND CORIANDER SALAD

1 tsp olive oil
1 tsp coriander seed
1 bay leaf
4 sprigs fresh parsley
1 stick celery, finely chopped
3 garlic cloves, crushed
½ tsp green peppercorns in brine
4 small fennel bulbs, trimmed and quartered
2 tbsp lemon juice
200ml/7fl oz white wine
200ml/7fl oz water
½ tsp sugar
Salt
1 bag mixed salad greens

Heat the oil, add the coriander seed and fry for a few minutes. Add the bay leaf, parsley, celery, garlic and peppercorns. Cook for 1 minute, then add the fennel, lemon juice, wine and water. Bring to the boil, add the sugar and a little salt, cover and simmer for 40 minutes. Drain the fennel, reserving the juices. Allow the fennel to cool slightly. Boil the juices rapidly to reduce a little.

Divide the salad greens between four plates, top with the fennel and pour over the juices.

SERVES: 4   CALORIES PER SERVING: 70   FAT: 3.4G

Nutrition notes: *Fennel is a mild diuretic and helpful in reducing water retention and improving digestion. Lemon juice is a good source of vitamin C.*

AUBERGINE PÂTÉ WITH GARLIC

1 large aubergine
2 tsp natural, unsweetened yogurt
2 tbsp chopped fresh parsley
1 tbsp chopped fresh chives
2 garlic cloves, crushed
4 tbsp lemon juice
Freshly ground black pepper
4 rye crispbreads
2 medium tomatoes

Cut the aubergine in half, lengthways. Place in the microwave oven and cook on High for 2 minutes, then turn and cook for another 2 minutes until soft. Scoop out the flesh, place in a piece of clean muslin or teatowel and squeeze gently to get rid of any bitter juices. Mash in a bowl with the yogurt, parsley, chives, garlic and lemon juice. Add black pepper to taste and serve with the crispbreads and sliced tomatoes.

SERVES: 4   CALORIES PER SERVING: 65   FAT: 1G

Nutrition notes: *Aubergines are high in potassium, but normal cooking methods involve frying, which makes them fat loaded. This recipe cuts the fat, and is a good way to boost your potassium intake if you're fed up with bananas!*

BRUSCHETTA WITH PARMESAN

An Italian favourite that's also a healthy, filling snack.

4 x 2.5cm/1in thick slices bread cut diagonally from a ciabatta or other Italian-style loaf
400g/14oz can chopped tomatoes
1 medium onion, finely chopped
2 cloves garlic, crushed
4 thin shavings Parmesan cheese
Flat-leaf parsley for garnish

Toast the bread on both sides. Meanwhile, empty the can of chopped tomatoes into a small pan, add the onion and garlic and cook briskly until reduced to a thick paste.

Top each slice of bread with the paste, a shaving of Parmesan cheese, and garnish with the parsley.

SERVES: 4   CALORIES PER SERVING: 90   FAT: 1G

Nutrition notes: *The bread is a good source of carbohydrates and the tomatoes contain some vitamin C. The garlic is good for lowering cholesterol and benefits the immune system. The Parmesan cheese contains protein, and just a little fat.*

PEPPER AND TOMATO GAZPACHO

This rich soup can be served warm or chilled, and if you prefer a chunkier soup, don't blend it.

2 large red peppers
1 large onion, chopped
2 sticks celery, trimmed and chopped
1 garlic clove, crushed
600ml/20fl oz vegetable stock
2 bay leaves
2 x 400g/14oz cans plum tomatoes
Pepper
2 spring onions, finely shredded
4 crispbreads for dunking

Preheat the grill. Halve and remove seeds from the peppers, arrange them on the grill and cook, turning occasionally, for 8–10 minutes until softened and charred. Leave to cool, then peel off the charred skin. Chop the pepper flesh and place in a large saucepan.

Stir in the onion, celery, garlic, stock and bay leaves. Bring to the boil, cover and simmer for 15 minutes. Remove from the heat.

Remove the bay leaves, stir in the tomatoes, and transfer to a blender. Blend until smooth, season with pepper, return to the pan and heat for 3–4 minutes until piping hot. Ladle into warm bowls and garnish with the spring onion. Serve with a crispbread for each person.

SERVES: 4   CALORIES PER PORTION (WITH CRISPBREAD): 100   FAT: 1G

Nutrition notes: *The peppers and tomatoes contain vitamin C and carbohydrate. Garlic benefits the heart and immune system. If you're exercising a lot, add some vermicelli pasta.*

Scrummy Snacks and Nibbles

SPICY STUFFED TOMATOES

4 large beefsteak tomatoes
2 tbsp fresh white breadcrumbs
2 tbsp chopped coriander
1 tbsp Worcestershire sauce
2 tsp chopped, crushed walnuts
½ tsp each curry powder and paprika
Coriander sprigs for decoration

Preheat oven to 180°C/350°F/Gas Mark 4. Cut the top third off each tomato and reserve as lids. Scoop out the seeds from each tomato and arrange, cut sides up, in an ovenproof dish. In a bowl, mix the breadcrumbs, coriander, Worcestershire sauce, crushed walnuts, curry powder and paprika. Stuff the tomatoes with the mixture, replace the lids, and bake in the oven for 15 minutes. Serve hot, garnished with coriander.

SERVES: 4   CALORIES PER SERVING: 90   FAT: 4.5G

Nutrition notes: *Tomatoes are an excellent source of vitamin C, betacarotene and other antioxidants which help to protect the body from the damaging effect of free radicals. Bread contains calcium as well as carbohydrates, and walnuts are rich in vegetable oils to protect your heart.*

RICE CAKE AND CRISPBREAD TOPPERS

These quick-to-prepare snacks are brilliant for preventing hunger pangs.

All under 100 calories, including base (about 30 cals)

Quorn Deli Slice, slice of beefsteak tomato
Cheese triangle, ½ tsp Marmite, celery, cucumber
2 tsp strawberry jam, 1 squirt aerosol cream or 2 tsp low-fat fromage frais
2 tsp lemon curd, sliced apricot or a few grapes
Thinly sliced apple, a few raisins, cinnamon and lemon juice to taste
2 tbsp cottage cheese with pineapple, slice of fresh orange, grapes to decorate
Small slice chicken, slice of mango
Slice of smoked salmon, cucumber and dill
2 tsp extra light soft cheese, sliced strawberries
1 tsp jam and 1 level tsp peanut butter

Nutrition notes: *All these snacks contain a nice mixture of protein (Quorn Deli Slices, cheese triangles, chicken, salmon, peanut butter) and carbs (tomato, jam, lemon curd, strawberries) to top up your daily intake.*

MERINGUE NEST TOPPERS

All under 100 calories (including the small meringue nest, 60 cals)

Slice of orange and 1 tsp Cointreau
2 slices kiwi fruit, sliced almond, a few raisins
6 raspberries, 1 squirt aerosol cream or 2 tsp low-fat fromage frais
2 tsp apricot jam, a few grapes
Half a 125g/4oz carton low-fat fruit yogurt, slice of orange
2 tsp canned fruit cocktail, squirt of aerosol cream
Small, sliced apple, sprinkling of cinnamon
2 tbsp low-fat cottage cheese, 3 sliced strawberries
2 tbsp low-fat fromage frais mixed with coffee flavouring to taste, sprinkled with 1 tsp grated chocolate
2 tsp vanilla ice-cream

86

MICROWAVED BANANAS WITH CINNAMON

4 small bananas
4 tsp ground cinnamon
Lemon juice to taste

Cut the banana skins lengthways along one side, very gently, without disturbing the fruit. Using the back of a teaspoon, rub 1 teaspoon cinnamon into each cut.

Place in the microwave and cook on High for about 30 seconds, until hot but not mushy. Sprinkle with lemon juice and enjoy!

SERVES: 4   CALORIES PER SERVING: 100   FAT: 0.7G

Nutrition notes: *Bananas contain carbohydrates, good levels of potassium and many vitamins. Ripe bananas are sweeter because more of their starch has been concentrated into sugar, but their calorie content is exactly the same as unripe bananas. Pre-exercise, it is better to eat a ripe banana as the sugar content has already been 'digested' and will provide a more rapid energy boost.*

87

ITALIAN RICE SALAD

This tasty salad is so low in calories that you could treat yourself to an extra portion.

400g/14oz can artichoke hearts
½ x 500g/17oz packet frozen peas and carrots
1 green pepper
1 yellow pepper
2 sticks celery
225g/8oz cold cooked long grain rice
400g/14oz can cooked button mushrooms, drained
100g/4oz can tuna in brine, drained and flaked
1 tbsp lemon juice
4 tbsp fat free salad dressing
Flat-leaf parsley or chives for garnish

Drain and rinse the artichoke hearts, and cut into pieces. Cook the frozen peas and carrots (or use leftovers), de-seed the peppers then dice. Chop the celery. Mix with the cold rice, then add the mushrooms, flaked tuna, lemon juice and dressing. Decorate with parsley or chives.

SERVES: 4   CALORIES PER SERVING: 95   FAT: 2G

Nutrition notes: *This salad contains a good selection of vegetables to add fibre, vitamins and minerals to the carb-rich rice base. It also contains protein (in tuna), vitamin C (lemon juice), vitamin A (carrots), and is very tasty too.*

SMOKED MACKEREL PÂTÉ

This is one of my favourite pâtés, and it is also great for parties.

225g/8oz smoked mackerel fillets, skinned, flaked and bones removed
125g/4oz very low-fat cheese spread or fromage frais
1 bunch watercress, leaves only, chopped
Finely grated zest and juice of ½ lime or lemon
Freshly ground black pepper

Mash the mackerel in a bowl and beat in the cheese spread or fromage frais. Stir in the watercress and lime or lemon zest, and add juice to taste. Season with pepper. Spoon into a serving dish, cover and refrigerate for at least 2 hours. Serve chilled, with crispbreads.

SERVES: 4   CALORIES PER SERVING (INCLUDING 1 CRISPBREAD): 160
FAT: 8.5G

Nutrition notes: *Mackerel is rich in omega-3 fatty acids which reduce blood cholesterol (their anti-inflammatory properties may also relieve arthritis). The watercress adds vitamin C.*

CHAPTER NINE

PERFECT PACKED LUNCHES

Gourmet meals to go

The best way to avoid those high street fast food fat traps and the equally fat-loaded fare in your office canteen or restaurant is to take a packed lunch to work or college. There is definitely something very satisfying (even smug!) about knowing that, deep in your workbag, there is a mini picnic of delicious sandwiches, home-made soup or fresh fruit salad just waiting to be gobbled up at lunch time.

By taking your own meal with you, you can avoid the daily grind of facing the crowds, queues and cash rip-offs that must be endured if you want to buy something decent to eat at midday. Instead, you can enjoy your spread at your leisure – in the park, at your desk or just sitting in the sunshine on a convenient bench while you watch the world go by.

One of the reasons I advise anyone who is trying to lose weight to eat a packed lunch is that preparing your own food gives you control over what you eat, and you decide on portion sizes. You don't even have to think about what the local burger bar has on offer, or worry about shelling out for a sad-looking tuna sandwich and overpriced cup of coffee. Your pre-packed meal can contain all the energizing, delicious, nutritious goodies that will help you get through the afternoon, yet be low in calories and fat – something that supermarket and fast food chains still find hard to achieve.

On the next few pages are some great ideas for packed meals, calorie and fat counted to help you plan your daily diet. They are also suitable for school children, so long as the rest of the kids' daily nutrient requirements are met (i.e. with additional protein, calcium and fibre). Quantities are for two (apart from the Apricot and Banana Compote, Hummus, Cheese Scones and Fruity Bread Pudding, which are best made in larger batches) so you can make enough for two days, or share your picnic with a mate.

To keep your feast fresh, pack salads in an air-tight container and use foil or cling film to protect solid items. Soups can be transported in a vacuum flask, and fruit should be washed and dried before packing in a paper bag.

CHICKEN AND HAM PÂTÉ WITH ORIENTAL SALAD

225g/8oz lean, cooked chicken (no skin)
100g/3½oz lean ham, trimmed of fat
Small bunch fresh parsley
1 garlic clove
1 tsp grated lime or lemon rind
2 tbsp lime or lemon juice
150g/5oz low-fat fromage frais
Salt and pepper
1 little gem lettuce
12 cherry tomatoes
2 kiwi fruit
1 banana
1 tbsp fat-free salad dressing

Finely chop the chicken and ham and place in a bowl. Chop the parsley and garlic and add to the meat. Add the lime or lemon rind and juice and fromage frais, and mix in gently. Season, cover and transfer to two airtight serving dishes (half for one day, half for the next).

To make the salad, separate the lettuce leaves, halve the tomatoes and peel and slice the kiwi fruit. Place in an airtight salad bowl. Pack in a picnic box, together with the banana and salad dressing (in a non-leak container), and 4 crispbreads. At lunchtime, slice the banana, toss with the salad and dressing, and eat with the pâté and crispbreads.

CALORIES PER SERVING: 350   FAT: 2.5G

Nutrition notes: *This pâté combines two good sources of protein, chicken and lean ham, with an excellent selection of other nutrients. The citrus juice contains vitamin C, the fromage frais contains calcium and the banana has carbohydrates and potassium. Together with the salad, this is a very well-balanced meal.*

BEAN AND VEGETABLE SOUP

Hot soups are always comforting, and this is especially heart-warming.

1 medium onion, chopped
1 garlic clove, finely chopped
2 celery sticks, sliced
1 large carrot, diced
400g/14oz can chopped tomatoes
150ml/5fl oz dry red wine
1.2 litres/2 pints vegetable stock
1 tsp dried oregano
425g/15oz can mixed beans (chickpea, kidney, cannellini etc.)
2 medium courgettes, diced
1 tbsp tomato purée
Salt and freshly ground black pepper

Place the onion, garlic, celery and carrot in a large saucepan. Stir in the tomatoes, red wine, vegetable stock and oregano. Bring the vegetable mixture to the boil, cover and leave to simmer for 15 minutes. Stir the beans and courgettes into the mixture and cook, uncovered, for 5 minutes.

Add the tomato purée to the mixture, and lightly season. Heat through and pour into a vacuum flask. Serve in a mug, with a medium crusty roll, and fruit to follow.

CALORIES PER SERVING: 320   FAT: 3G

Nutrition notes: *Beans are a valuable source of protein, B vitamins, iron and fibre. Garlic helps ward off infection and lowers cholesterol, and the wine adds a real kick. It is a bulky soup, so if you add some fruit and a roll, you will feel very full up indeed.*

CURRIED CHICKEN BREASTS WITH SPICY CARROT DIP

The ubiquitous high-protein, low-fat chicken breast is given a new, sexy taste with this delicious curry recipe.

CURRIED CHICKEN BREASTS:

4 x 125g/4½oz boneless, skinless chicken breasts
1 garlic clove, crushed
2.5cm/1in piece root ginger, finely chopped
1 fresh green chilli, seeded and finely chopped
6 tbsp low-fat natural yogurt
1 tbsp tomato purée
1 tsp ground turmeric
1 tsp garam masala
1 tbsp lime juice
Freshly ground black pepper

SPICY CARROT DIP:

1 medium onion
3 medium carrots
Grated rind and juice of 2 oranges
1 tbsp hot curry paste
150g/5oz low-fat natural yogurt
Small handful fresh basil leaves
2 tbsp lemon juice
Tabasco to taste
A little salt and freshly ground black pepper

First, cook the chicken. Preheat the oven to 190°C/375°F/Gas Mark 5. In a small bowl, mix together the garlic, ginger, chilli, yogurt, tomato purée, turmeric, garam masala, lime juice and seasoning. Wash and pat dry the chicken breasts, place on a baking sheet and spread the spicy mixture over the top. Bake for 30–35 minutes, until meat is tender and cooked through.

Meanwhile, make the dip. Finely chop the onion, grate the carrots, and mix together in a small saucepan with the orange rind and juice and hot curry paste. Bring to the boil, cover and simmer for about 10 minutes. Leave to cool, then stir in the yogurt, chopped basil leaves, lemon juice, Tabasco and seasoning to taste.

Wrap cold chicken in foil, and put the dip in an airtight container to transport. This is great with a simple green salad and kiwi fruit to follow.

CALORIES PER PORTION – CHICKEN: 350 (2 CHICKEN BREASTS PER PERSON). DIP: 60

FAT – CHICKEN: 4G   DIP: 0.5G

Nutrition notes: *Garlic, ginger and chilli have anti-infection properties, and are thought to enhance sexual prowess. The carrot dip provides vitamin A, important for healthy eyes, and kiwi is a good source of vitamin C. So this is an excellent lunch if you are working in front of a computer all day and are planning a romantic evening!*

STUFFED PEPPERS WITH CREAMY COLESLAW

These peppers are also good served hot as an accompaniment to grilled fish or cold meat.

STUFFED PEPPERS:
50g/2oz brown or white rice
2 red peppers
185g/6oz can tuna in brine, drained and flaked
2 tbsp canned sweetcorn kernals, drained
1 tbsp dry white breadcrumbs
1 tbsp grated Parmesan cheese
Basil or parsley leaves to garnish

CREAMY COLESLAW:
½ small head white cabbage, thinly sliced
1 medium carrot, grated
2 tbsp raisins
150g/5oz carton cottage cheese with chives
1 tbsp low-calorie mayonnaise
Freshly ground black pepper

Cook the rice in plenty of water (it should be firm, not mushy), drain and place in a bowl. Preheat the grill to medium. Halve the peppers, remove the seeds and stalks and grill, cut-side down, for 5 minutes. Turn and cook for a further 5 minutes.

Add the tuna and sweetcorn to the rice in the bowl, season and use to fill the four pepper halves. Mix together the breadcrumbs and grated Parmesan cheese. Sprinkle over the top, and place the peppers back under the grill for 4–5 minutes until hot and golden brown. Allow to cool, and pack in an airtight container.

Fight Fat, Fight Fatigue Diet and Cookbook

Mix the cabbage, carrot and raisins in a plastic, airtight bowl. Mix the cottage cheese, mayonnaise and seasoning and put in a separate airtight bowl. Just before eating, mix the two together.

CALORIES PER SERVING: 250   FAT: 4.2G

Nutrition notes: *Red peppers are a very rich source of vitamin C, and if you choose brown instead of white rice you will get extra fibre in this dish. The coleslaw is much healthier than the shop-bought kind (and lower in calories) because the raisins add inositol (a member of the vitamin B group) and the cottage cheese adds calcium and vitamin D.*

APRICOT AND BANANA COMPOTE

This is delicious for breakfast as well as lunch, and it is also good served hot. Kids love it!

225g/8oz dried apricots
300ml/10fl oz unsweetened orange juice
150ml/5fl oz unsweetened apple juice
1 tsp ground ginger
3 medium bananas, sliced
25g/1oz toasted flaked almonds

Put the apricots in a saucepan with the fruit juices and ginger, and stir. Cover, bring to the boil and simmer gently for 10 minutes, stirring occasionally. Leave to cool, then pack a quarter of the mixture in an airtight bowl, with the almonds packed in foil. Mix the sliced bananas and almonds into the compote just before eating.

SERVES: 4   CALORIES PER SERVING: 240   FAT: 4.2G

Nutrition notes: *Dried apricots are rich in betacarotene, which has antioxidant properties, yet low in calories (about 10 cals each). The bananas supply carbohydrate, and the flaked almonds contain protein and a little fat.*

DOUBLE-DECKER SANDWICH

Double-decker sandwiches make a filling lunch, but are usually calorie-loaded. By making them yourself, you can reduce the calorie and fat content.

6 slices wholemeal bread
50g/2oz sliced cooked cold meat (eg. tongue, lean ham) or Quorn slices
2 gherkins, chopped
2 tbsp sweetcorn
1 tsp low-calorie mayonnaise
1 stick celery
1 small dessert apple
2 tsp lemon juice
12g/½oz chopped nuts

99

Arrange the cooked meat on two slices of bread, and top with the gherkins, sweetcorn and mayonnaise. Cover with two more slices of bread, then top with chopped celery, apple, lemon juice and nuts and the final two slices of bread. Cut each double-decker sandwich in half diagonally and wrap in foil or cling film.

CALORIES PER SANDWICH: 345   FAT: 3G

Nutrition notes: *Using wholemeal bread for your double-decker sarnie gives you valuable fibre and vitamin B. It is also a 'slow-release' carb, so it provides longer-lasting energy than white bread. Making one filling meat-based (providing protein) and the other veggie-based (providing carbs, minerals, vitamins) gives a well-balanced 'meal' in one sandwich.*

CHINESE SALAD WITH YOGURT DRESSING

Water chestnuts add a crunch to this simple yet unusual salad. The dressing is scrumptious.

SALAD:
25g/1oz toasted hazelnuts
75g/3oz grapes, halved and seeded if necessary
50g/2oz canned water chestnuts, drained
100g/4oz Chinese leaves, finely shredded
225g/8oz bite-sized pieces cooked turkey meat (or Quorn slices)

DRESSING:
1 tsp grated Parmesan cheese
1 tsp olive oil
1 tsp lemon juice
Small pinch English mustard powder
1 garlic clove, crushed
Few drops Worcestershire or light soy sauce
150g/5oz unsweetened natural yogurt

Combine the salad ingredients and put in a plastic bowl with an air-tight lid. Whisk together the first six dressing ingredients, then stir in the yogurt. Pack in a screw-top jar and shake before pouring over the salad.

CALORIES PER SERVING: 420   FAT: 5.3G

Nutrition notes: *Hazelnuts are rich in vegetable oils and protein, and the cooked turkey is also a good source of protein. There is just enough cheese to give piquancy to the dressing without adding too much fat, and the yogurt adds valuable calcium to help build strong bones.*

LOW-FAT HUMMUS WITH PITTA AND SALAD

175g/6oz canned chickpeas (reserve the liquid)
3 tbsp sesame seeds
2 garlic cloves
2 tbsp lemon juice
1 tsp ground coriander
1 tbsp fat-free vinaigrette dressing (Kraft)
Pinch each salt and pepper
175g/6oz low-fat soft cheese spread

TO SERVE:
4 pitta breads
Mixed vegetable salad

Place all the hummus ingredients in a blender, add a little of the
chickpea liquid and blend until smooth. Serve with 1 pitta bread per
person, and a mixed vegetable salad (eg. carrot, cucumber, celery),
packed in suitable containers.

101

CALORIES PER SERVING: 265   FAT: 3.5G

Nutrition notes: *Shop-bought hummus is usually very high in calories, so this simple
recipe is very useful for slimmers. It is also very nutritious as chickpeas (and other pulses
such as butter and kidney beans) are full of protein and fibre, and lemon juice provides
vitamin C. The low-fat soft cheese is good, too – containing valuable calcium and
vitamin D.*

HOME-MADE SCONES WITH CHEESE FILLING

125g/4oz plain flour
3½ tsp baking powder
¼ tsp powdered mustard
Pinch of salt
4 tbsp low-fat margarine
90g/3oz low-fat Cheddar cheese, finely grated
2 tbsp chopped chives
200ml/7fl oz skimmed milk

FILLING:
125g/4oz low-fat soft cheese
250g/9oz low-fat fromage frais
Dash of Tabasco

Line 2 baking sheets with non-stick baking parchment. Reserve one tablespoon flour and sift the remainder into a large bowl with the baking powder, mustard and salt. Rub the margarine into the flour mixture. Stir in the grated cheese and chives. Add enough milk to form a soft dough. Sprinkle the remaining flour on a work surface, and gently knead the dough. Roll out the dough until about 2cm/ ¾ in thick. Cut into 12 rounds and leave to stand at room temperature for 10 minutes.

Bake in a preheated oven at 210°C/425°F/Gas Mark 7 for 12–15 minutes. Cool on a wire rack. Mix the soft cheese and fromage frais, and add Tabasco to taste. Split the scones and spread with the mixture.

MAKES: 12   CALORIES PER FILLED SCONE: 195   FAT: 4.5G

Nutrition notes: *These are good for the family as they are filling, and the cheesy spread boosts the calcium content. However, beware of eating too many.*

Fight Fat, Fight Fatigue Diet and Cookbook

FRUITY BREAD PUDDING

This traditional dish is delicious hot or cold. When cold, it is very easy
to pack in greaseproof paper.

6 medium slices stale wholemeal bread
50g/2oz strawberry jam or lemon curd
A little low-fat spread to grease dish
50g/2oz sultanas
50g/2oz dried apricots, chopped
5og/2oz soft light brown sugar
1 tsp ground mixed spice
2 eggs
600ml/20fl oz skimmed milk
Finely grated rind of 1 lemon

Preheat the oven to 160°C/325°F/Gas Mark 3. Cut the crusts off the
bread, spread each slice with jam or lemon curd and cut into four
triangles. Lightly grease a shallow, rectangular ovenproof dish and
place half the triangles in it. Mix the sultanas, apricots, sugar and
spice and sprinkle half this mixture over the bread in the dish. Top
with the remaining bread triangles and fruit. Beat the eggs, milk and
lemon rind together and pour over the bread and fruit. Set aside for
about 20 minutes, then bake for 45–60 minutes until lightly set and
golden.

SERVES: 4   CALORIES PER SERVING: 300   FAT: 4.5G.

Nutrition notes: *The bread is fibre-rich and filling, and the apricots add
betacarotene to the dish. The eggs provide iron and protein and the skimmed milk
supplies calcium.*

CHAPTER TEN

FAMILY SUPPER DISHES

Filling dishes for hungry customers

You're harassed, tired and there's nothing in the fridge. Help! The easiest thing in the world is to go to the freezer, pick out a ready meal plus some frozen veg, and serve a quick supper. The only problem? Frankly, 'instant' suppers are boring, don't contain enough essential nutrients to keep you and your family in tip-top good health, and they encourage weight gain because they leave your taste-buds and tummy feeling cheated, so you can't resist some tasty chocs or crisps during the evening.

It's just as easy to serve up something fresh, delicious and nutritious that is low in calories and fat, and is suitable for the whole family. What's more, it's often quicker as well. Over the years I have learned that 'convenience food' is often far from convenient. By the time you've broken a nail trying to undo the fiddly packaging, searched the kitchen for scissors to snip open the various sachets inside, and heated it all up in two different pans, you could easily have made a delicious omelette or grilled a steak and whizzed up some salad.

The 10 recipes in this chapter are simple to make, yet each dish contains a cocktail of the brilliant, hard-working nutrients you need to prevent tiredness and help you get slim and fit. They are also packed with fibre, vitamins and minerals, and low-fat protein.

I haven't completely ignored packaged foods, either: to my mind the most useful store cupboard basics are canned and bottled foods like chopped tomatoes, tuna, beans, anchovies, artichoke hearts, bottled chillies and oriental sauces. My freezer is full of my own dishes, meat, fish and desserts, but I do confess that I also have frozen peas, sweetcorn and green beans in case my local greengrocer is closed.

After eating one of these suppers, you will notice that you feel less tired, happier and less inclined to snack in the evenings. What's more, kids will be less tetchy than they are on a diet of ready meals and takeaways.

All recipes serve four, and seven of the choices are either suitable for vegetarians or can be adapted for vegetarians.

CHICKEN MARYLAND

4 frozen sweetcorn cobs
4 boneless chicken breasts (preferably free-range)
Salt and black pepper
A little corn or olive oil for brushing
225g/8oz lean rindless, unsmoked bacon
4 ripe bananas, peeled and halved
4 firm large tomatoes, halved
1 crisp lettuce, torn into large pieces
1 bunch watercress
Freshly ground black pepper

DRESSING:
2 tsp honey
1 tbsp white wine vinegar
2 tsp Dijon mustard

Bring a large pan of water to the boil. Boil the sweetcorn for 15 minutes, then drain. Season the chicken breasts, brush with oil and grill for 15 minutes, turning once. Grill the bacon until crisp, and the bananas, tomatoes and sweetcorn until lightly browned. Combine the lettuce and watercress. Place the dressing ingredients in a jar, shake, and then toss the salad greens with the dressing.

To serve, place salad greens on four plates and top with the chicken, tomato, sweetcorn, bacon and banana.

CALORIES PER SERVING: 490   FAT: 5G

Nutrition notes: *Chicken is a good protein source, bacon and watercress provide iron, sweetcorn provides betacarotene and tomatoes contain vitamin C. Bananas contain carbohydrates and potassium.*

Fight Fat, Fight Fatigue Diet and Cookbook

POLYNESIAN BEEF STIR-FRY

200g/7oz can bamboo shoots
1 beef stock cube
2 tsp oil
1 large onion, chopped
1 tbsp grated fresh ginger
225g/8oz rump steak (or you could use pork tenderloin – or Quorn pieces if you are vegetarian), very thinly sliced
1 tsp cornflour
1 tbsp dry sherry
2 tbsp soy sauce
425g/15oz can red kidney beans, drained
Freshly ground black pepper
Sliced lemon, radish and watercress for garnish

Drain the liquid from the bamboo shoots into a small pan, heat and dissolve the stock cube in the liquid. Heat the oil in a wok or large shallow non-stick pan and gently fry the onion and ginger until the onion is transparent. Push to one side of the pan and add the beef. Stir-fry briskly until the meat is sealed.

Mix the cornflour with the sherry and soy sauce and add to the pan with the bamboo shoots, drained beans and stock. Stir gently, cook for one minute, season to taste, and serve on hot plates garnished with the lemon, radish and watercress, plus wholegrain rice, noodles or pasta and a large salad.

CALORIES PER SERVING: 160   FAT: 3G

Nutrition notes: *Red meat is an important source of iron and protein. Kidney beans are also protein-rich and a good source of fibre. Ginger is a good cold preventative, and excellent for the circulation.*

Family Supper Dishes

LOW-FAT MOUSSAKA

A crisp Greek salad would be tasty with this.

450g/1lb lean minced beef or lamb (or Quorn pieces)
1 large onion, chopped
1 large aubergine, sliced
150g/6oz courgettes, sliced
400g/14oz can chopped tomatoes with garlic and herbs
2 tsp gravy browning granules
150g/6oz potatoes, par-boiled and sliced
1 packet white sauce mix
300ml/10fl oz skimmed milk
50g/2oz low-fat Cheddar-type cheese

Brown the mince in a large non-stick saucepan. Remove with a slotted spoon and drain on kitchen paper. Place onion, aubergine and courgette slices in a pan with the tomatoes. Add the mince, bring to the boil, then lower the temperature and cook gently for 30 minutes. Add browning granules, stir and cook for a further minute. Place in an ovenproof dish, and top with the potatoes. Make up the sauce mix with the milk, grate in the cheese, and pour over the top of the potatoes.

Bake in a preheated oven at 190°C/375°F/Gas Mark 5 for about 30 minutes or until the top is browned. You can make this dish up to 48 hours in advance, and it will freeze for up to three months.

CALORIES PER PORTION: 350   FAT: 10G

Nutrition notes: *Lean mince is a good protein source and a better buy than cheaper, fattier meat because it goes further. The vegetables add fibre to the basic dish, and the milk and cheese provide valuable calcium.*

NORMANDY PORK

8 lean pork medallions or tenderloin steaks, about 50g/1¾ oz each
2 tsp olive oil
1 medium onion, finely sliced
1 tsp caster sugar
1 tsp dried sage
150ml/5fl oz dry cider
150ml/5fl oz chicken stock
1 green and 1 red apple
1 tbsp lemon juice
Salt and freshly ground black pepper
4 tbsp natural yogurt or fromage frais and fresh sage leaves for garnish

Trim away any excess fat from the meat. Heat the oil in a non-stick pan and gently fry the onion for 5 minutes until softened. Add the sugar and cook gently for 3–4 minutes until golden. Add the pork to the pan and cook for 2 minutes on each side until browned. Add the dried sage, cider and stock. Bring to the boil, cover, and simmer gently for 20 minutes until the pork is cooked. Meanwhile, core and cut each apple into 8 wedges and toss in lemon juice to prevent browning.

Add the apples to the pork, mix gently, season lightly and cook for 2–4 minutes until the apple wedges are tender. Serve with a tablespoon of yogurt or fromage frais and a sprig of sage on top of each pork medallion or steak.

CALORIES PER SERVING: 200   FAT: 6G

Nutrition notes: *If you trim off the fat, pork is as low in calories as chicken, and is an excellent source of protein and B vitamins. However, it is not as rich in iron as other red meats. The apples supply fibre, potassium and vitamin C and the yogurt adds calcium.*

LOWER FAT ORIENTAL STIR-FRY

This adaptable recipe can include meat, fish or vegetarian protein. You could also adapt it to include crunchy vegetables such as cauliflower, sliced fennel and carrots. Serve with noodles or boiled rice.

125g/4oz broccoli florets
4 spring onions
1 tsp cornflour
3 tbsp oyster sauce
1 tbsp dark soy sauce
120ml/4fl oz chicken or vegetable stock
2 tsp lemon juice
3 tsp olive oil
1 small onion, chopped
2 garlic cloves, crushed
2 tsp grated fresh root ginger
450g/1lb turkey steaks or chicken breasts, cut into small pieces; or Quorn pieces or tofu, cut into chunks; or defrosted frozen cooked prawns or squid; or firm fish, cut into pieces
125g/4oz mushrooms (shiitake if possible), sliced
75g/3oz baby sweetcorn, halved lengthways
Salt and freshly ground black pepper
Shredded spring onion or fresh coriander to garnish

Divide the broccoli florets into sprigs and cut the stalks into thin, diagonal slices. Finely chop the white parts of the spring onions and slice the green parts. In a bowl, blend together the cornflour, oyster sauce, soy sauce, stock and lemon juice.

Heat the olive oil in a wok or non-stick pan. Add the onion, garlic and ginger and stir-fry for a minute, then add the meat, Quorn, tofu or fish, and stir-fry for 2 minutes, until cooked. Remove from the wok with a slotted spoon and keep warm.

Add the broccoli, mushrooms and sweetcorn to the pan with a little of the sauce to prevent sticking. Stir-fry briskly for 2 minutes. Return the meat, Quorn, tofu or fish to the wok and add the chopped spring onion and the rest of the sauce. Stir for about 1 minute, until the sauce has thickened. Serve garnished with spring onion or coriander.

CALORIES PER SERVING: 230   FAT: 6G

Nutrition notes: *This is a very healthy stir-fry with a good selection of nutrients – the basic ingredient (whether it is meat, fish or one of the veggie alternatives) provides protein, while broccoli is a useful source of both vitamin C and betacarotene, which are powerful antioxidants and can help protect us from heart disease and some cancers.*

111

LEEK AND SEAFOOD LASAGNE

If you're vegetarian, substitute tofu, Quorn pieces or hard-boiled egg quarters for the seafood. This dish goes well with a tomato and cucumber salad.

450g/1lb leeks
150ml/5fl oz vegetable stock or water
A little cornflour
Freshly ground black pepper
Grated nutmeg
450g/1lb smoked haddock fillet
300ml/10fl oz skimmed milk
1 packet savoury white sauce mix
2 tsp freshly chopped dill or parsley
100g/4oz peeled prawns (or 450g/1lb tofu or Quorn pieces, or hard-boiled egg quarters)
150g/5oz quick-cook lasagne
1 egg
150g/5oz carton low-fat natural yogurt
3 tbsp grated Parmesan cheese

Trim, clean and slice the leeks and simmer in the vegetable stock or water until tender, about 10 minutes. Thicken the cooking liquor to the consistency of fairly runny sauce using a little cornflour. Season to taste with the pepper and grated nutmeg.

Cut the smoked haddock into bite-size pieces and simmer in the skimmed milk for about 5 minutes. Drain the fish, reserving the milk. (If you're making the veggie option leave out this part and simply add your tofu etc. to the sauce.)

Make up the sauce mix with the milk (it should be quite runny) and season. Stir in the dill, prawns and haddock (or veggie substitutes).

Preheat the oven to 190°C/375°F/Gas Mark 5. Put a layer of lasagne into the bottom of an ovenproof dish. Spoon on the leeks, then add another layer of lasagne and the fish or veggie mixture. Top with a final layer of lasagne. Beat the egg with the yogurt, stir in the Parmesan, season and pour over the top. Bake in the preheated oven for about 40 minutes until browned and bubbling. Serve immediately.

CALORIES PER SERVING: 340   FAT: 4G

Nutrition notes: *Pasta is carb-rich to help 'fuel' muscles. The smoked haddock supplies protein but it is quite high in salt, so don't include any salt in the seasoning if you're using fish. Leeks have lots of potassium and are a good diuretic, helping to relieve water retention. Instead of leeks you could use spinach – another nutritionally valuable vegetable.*

113

MIXED STUFFED VEGETABLES

4 large beefsteak tomatoes
4 large courgettes
2 red peppers
225g/8oz cracked wheat
¼ cucumber
1 medium red onion
2 tbsp lemon juice
2 tbsp chopped fresh coriander
2 tbsp chopped fresh mint
1 tbsp olive oil
2 tsp cumin seeds
3 tbsp chopped, leftover cooked meat or fish, or chickpeas

Preheat the oven to 200°C/400°F/Gas Mark 6. Cut off the tops of the tomatoes and reserve. Scoop out the pulp, chop and place in a bowl. Trim the courgettes and cut a V-shaped groove down each one. Finely chop the cut-out courgette flesh and add to the tomato pulp. Halve the peppers, leaving the stalks intact, and cut out the seeds.

Soak the cracked wheat according to the instructions on the packet. Finely chop the cucumber and red onion and add to the tomato pulp and courgette mixture. Mix the wheat, lemon juice, coriander, mint, olive oil and cumin seeds with the vegetables and meat or chickpeas. Stuff the mixture into the vegetable shells. Place the tops on the tomatoes, transfer to a roasting tin and bake for 20–25 minutes until cooked through.

CALORIES PER SERVING: 400   FAT: 6.5G

Nutrition notes: *The courgettes are a good carbohydrate source and have more fibre when baked than boiled, and the cracked wheat has valuable B vitamins and vitamin E.*

PLAICE WITH MUSTARD SAUCE

This is a quick, tasty way of preparing any white fish fillets. It's perfect as a low-calorie lunch, as well as for supper.

4 plaice or flounder fillets (or any filleted white fish or Quorn steaks)
1 tsp olive oil
2 shallots, chopped
2 tbsp Dijon mustard
150g/5oz low-fat crème fraîche or fromage frais
Watercress

Preheat the oven to 180°C/350°F/Gas Mark 4. Brush a shallow ovenproof dish with the oil and place the fish fillets in the dish. Mix the shallots, mustard and low-fat crème fraîche or fromage frais together and pour over the fish. Bake in the oven for 15–20 minutes. Serve with watercress.

CALORIES PER SERVING: 200   FAT: 3G

Nutrition notes: *Plaice is an excellent source of protein, and is low in calories and fat. It also contains B vitamins and minerals such as iodine and selenium. The crème fraîche or fromage frais is a good, low-fat source of calcium.*

PANCAKES WITH RICOTTA CHEESE AND SPINACH

Although still fairly high in fat (make sure you eat 'lean' for the rest of the day!), these pancakes are much lower in fat than the usual kind, as they contain skimmed milk instead of whole milk.

BATTER:
150ml/5fl oz skimmed milk
175ml/6fl oz soda water
Pinch of salt
125g/4oz strong white plain flour, sifted
1 egg
25g/1oz butter or 2 tsp olive oil

FILLING:
225g/8oz fresh or frozen spinach
400g/14oz ricotta cheese
1 size 1 egg, lightly beaten
½ tsp grated lemon rind
½ tsp ground cinnamon
½ tsp salt
Freshly ground black pepper
1 tbsp chopped fresh chives, for garnish

Heat the oven to 180°C/350°F/Gas Mark 4. To make the pancakes (easier than it sounds!): combine the milk, soda water and salt in a jug. Place the flour and egg in a large bowl and beat vigorously, adding the milk and water mixture little by little until you have a smooth, creamy texture. Set aside for 30 minutes (or make earlier in the day and keep in the fridge until needed).

Smear a non-stick frying pan with just enough butter or oil to gloss the surface. Place on a hot gas ring or electric plate, and when the pan is very hot pour in ⅛ of the batter. Tilt the pan to spread it. Cook for 1 minute, then flip with a palette knife or spatula and cook the other side for 1 minute (if you are nervous about turning the pancake over, brown the top under a hot grill instead). Cook seven more pancakes the same way. The pancakes can be cooked in advance and stored in the fridge, or frozen (place a piece of foil between each one to avoid sticking.

To make the filling, wash and trim fresh spinach, wring it out very thoroughly, squeezing out as much of the liquid as you can, then chop and mix it with the cheese. (If you are using frozen spinach, allow it to defrost, then squeeze out the water and mix with the cheese). Add the egg, lemon rind, cinnamon, salt and pepper and mix thoroughly.

Spread some of the mixture over each pancake, roll up and place, seam down, in a shallow ovenproof dish. If you have mixture leftover, spread it along the centre of the row of pancakes. Bake in the preheated oven for about 20 minutes.

CALORIES PER PORTION: 330   FAT: 18G

Nutrition notes: *Skimmed milk is a good source of calcium. The flour supplies carbohydrate to fuel muscles, and the filling is rich in calcium (cheese) and antioxidants (spinach).*

BEEF CASSEROLE WITH GUINNESS

675g/1½lb very lean, cubed stewing steak
2 tsp olive oil
350g/12oz onions
350g/12oz carrots, peeled and roughly chopped
4 sticks celery, chopped
1 garlic clove, crushed
330ml bottle Guinness Extra
3 tbsp tomato purée
Freshly ground black pepper to taste
A little water
Freshly ground black pepper
Chopped parsley

118

Heat the oil until hot in a large, cast iron casserole. Brown the meat, one layer at a time. Using a slotted spoon, transfer each batch onto a side plate. Peel and coarsely chop the onions and brown these as well, transferring to the same plate with a slotted spoon. Pour off the excess fat in the casserole. Return meat and onions to the pan, add the carrots, celery, garlic, Guinness and tomato purée. Season with pepper, bring to the boil, then turn the heat right down, cover and leave to simmer for about 2 hours. Alternatively, place the casserole in a moderate (180°C/350°F/Gas Mark 4) oven for about 2 hours.

During cooking, check the casserole every so often, scraping the bottom and adding a little water as the gravy thickens. When the meat is tender, check the seasoning, and garnish with freshly chopped parsley. Serve straight from the casserole. This freezes well.

CALORIES PER SERVING: 270   FAT: 9.5G

Nutrition notes: *Beef is very high in protein, B vitamins, iron and zinc, and Guinness is also mineral-rich. The fat content of the dish is minimized by using lean beef.*

Fight Fat, Fight Fatigue Diet and Cookbook

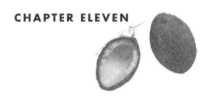

CHAPTER ELEVEN

DINNER PARTY DISHES

Cheat's guide to impressing your guests

There is a (very plausible) theory around that the popularity of cookery programmes on TV has nothing to do with people actually wanting to learn how to cook. The real reason viewers switch on to watch the latest celebrity chef showing off his or her skills is to salivate over the amazingly fattening ingredients they use in almost every dish.

After the viewers' taste buds have been tickled to death and they've worked up a good appetite they are inspired, not to create their own culinary masterpiece, but to phone for a pizza.

Frankly, I am appalled by the vast amounts of double cream, butter and cheese, and great slurps of olive oil that seem to be essential for every dish produced by TV chefs. With the current obesity crisis causing so much concern, it would be more helpful if they showed the public how to produce delicious meals that don't rely on high-fat ingredients. You simply don't have to overload dishes with fat to produce a tasty result: for instance, you can swap double cream for low-fat fromage frais in many recipes, limit olive oil to the amount really needed (usually half the amount given in a recipe), use low-fat soft cheese in place of the full-fat kind and filo pastry instead of fat-loaded shortcrust. It's so lazy, I feel, to carry on using harmful quantities of fat when it is totally unnecessary.

It really is quite easy to produce brilliant dishes which are healthy as well. To prove it, I've come up with these starters, main courses and puds which are special enough to dish up for guests, yet surprisingly low in calories and fat. They also supply a great variety of essential nutrients which will help you look and feel terrific. Incorporated into your diet plan, these recipes will convince you that staying in shape doesn't have to be dull. All the recipes serve four, with the exception of the Dinner Party Gateau.

STARTERS

BORSCHT WITH CAVIAR

450g/1lb cooked beetroot (not in vinegar)
1 medium onion
600ml/20fl oz beef stock, fresh or from a cube
2 tbsp freshly chopped dill
Salt and freshly ground pepper
Lemon juice and a little sugar to taste
4 tbsp low-fat natural yogurt
4 tbsp caviar or black lumpfish roe

Chop the beetroot into small pieces and chop the onion very finely. Place in a blender or food processor with the stock. Liquidize and add herbs and seasoning to taste. Add lemon juice and sugar to taste – the juice of half a lemon, plus half a teaspoon of sugar should be just about right. If necessary, thin the soup with a little more water or stock and chill well.

Pour into individual bowls and top each with a swirl of yogurt and a teaspoon of caviar. This can be made the day before your party, with the garnish added on the day.

CALORIES PER SERVING: 90   FAT: 2G

Nutrition notes: *Beetroot contains folic acid, one of the B group of vitamins which is important for healthy blood cells and vital for women during pregnancy. So if you are a mum-to-be and develop a craving for this delicious soup – indulge. Beetroot is also a good source of fibre. Yogurt provides calcium, and caviar contains omega-3 fatty acids which can help prevent heart disease.*

ORIENTAL FISH SALAD

Vegetarians could top this salad with spicy beans mixed with the onions, chillies and pineapple instead of the fish.

225g/8oz trout fillets
225g/8oz haddock or cod fillets
300ml/10fl oz water
1 stalk lemon grass
2 lime leaves or 1 small lime, sliced
1 large red fresh chilli or 2 small canned chillies
Bunch spring onions, trimmed and shredded
1 small red pepper, seeded and diced
125g/4oz fresh or canned pineapple, diced
1 bunch watercress, trimmed
Fresh chives for garnish

DRESSING:
2 tbsp fat-free vinaigrette dressing
Pinch of chilli powder
1 tsp clear honey
Freshly ground black pepper

Rinse the fish and place in a frying pan with the water, bruised lemon grass (bend it in half to bruise it), lime leaves or sliced lime. Prick the chilli with a fork and add to the pan. Bring to the boil and simmer for 7–8 minutes. Allow to cool. Drain the fish and flake the flesh. Place the flaked fish in a bowl and gently stir in the spring onions, red pepper and pineapple.

Arrange the watercress on 4 plates and top with the cooked fish mixture. Mix the dressing ingredients together, season with pepper and spoon over the fish. Garnish with chopped chives.

CALORIES PER SERVING: 180   FAT: 4G

Nutrition notes: *Fish is an excellent source of protein and the oily trout has omega-3 fatty acids to help keep your heart healthy. Lime and red pepper both contain vitamin C, and watercress is a super source of antioxidants – especially betacarotene. It also has iron and calcium, plus fibre. Pineapple is good for digestion and contains vitamin C, manganese and potassium. This starter will do your guests a power of good.*

123

STUFFED COURGETTES

This could be served as a lunch dish, too, with a jacket potato to provide extra carbs and fibre.

8 medium courgettes
1 tsp oil
1 garlic clove, finely chopped
400g/14oz can chopped tomatoes
50g/2oz can anchovies, well drained
1 tsp dried or fresh marjoram or basil, chopped
Freshly ground black pepper

Preheat the oven to 200°C/400°F/Gas Mark 6. Slice the courgettes in half lengthways, scoop out the seeds and seed pulp and discard. Heat the oil in a saucepan and lightly fry the garlic. Add the chopped tomatoes, bring to the boil and cook on high heat until the tomatoes are reduced by about half. Remove from the heat and stir in one chopped anchovy fillet and half the marjoram or basil.

Wipe the insides of the courgettes with a paper towel, and place in a large baking dish. Fill each one with tomato sauce and arrange the remaining anchovy fillets on top. Grind over plenty of black pepper and bake for about 35 minutes until tender. Allow to cool before serving, sprinkled with the remaining herbs.

CALORIES PER SERVING: 50   FAT: 2.75G

Nutrition notes: *This very low-calorie starter is surprisingly nutritious – courgettes contain fibre and minerals, tomatoes are rich in vitamin C, and anchovies contain fish oils, which are good for the heart.*

PEARS ROQUEFORT

This would also make a delicious lunch dish, served with a larger, mixed salad.

50g/2oz Roquefort cheese
125g/4oz very low-fat soft cheese
Pinch of white pepper
1 tsp paprika
2 large, ripe pears
1–2 tbsp lemon juice
Mixed salad leaves (eg. rocket, lamb's lettuce, radicchio)
6 tbsp oil-free dressing
Extra paprika for garnish

Mash the two cheeses together, and season with the pepper and paprika. Peel, halve and core the pears and paint with lemon juice to prevent discolouring. Fill the core cavities with about two thirds of the cheese mixture.

Arrange the salad leaves on four small plates. Top each with a pear half, cut side down. Now blend the rest of the cheese mixture with the oil-free dressing, and spoon over the pears. Sprinkle with paprika and serve immediately.

CALORIES PER SERVING: 100   FAT: 4.75G

Nutrition notes: *Roquefort is lower in fat than other blue cheeses. Its flavour is also strong enough that you need only a little, so the calorie content of this dish is considerably lowered. Pears are a good source of vitamins, minerals and fibre, and, of course, the cheese supplies calcium.*

MAIN COURSES

GINGER BEEF STEAKS WITH PINEAPPLE SALSA

4 lean fillet or rump steaks about 100g/3½ oz each, trimmed of fat
Freshly ground black pepper
2 tbsp ginger wine
2.5cm/1in piece root ginger, finely chopped
2 garlic cloves, crushed
1 tsp chilli powder
1 tsp olive oil
Red chilli strips for garnish

SALSA:
225g/8oz fresh or canned pineapple, chopped
1 small red pepper, halved, seeded and finely chopped
2 tbsp light soy sauce
1 piece stem ginger in syrup, drained and chopped

Pound the steaks with a mallet or rolling pin until 1cm/½ inch thick. Season with pepper and place in a shallow dish. Mix the wine, ginger, garlic and chilli powder and pour over the meat. Chill for 30 minutes.

Mix the salsa ingredients together, cover and chill. Brush a grill pan or heavy frying pan with the olive oil, and heat well. Drain the beef and add to the pan. Lower the heat and cook the steaks for 10 minutes, turning once. Drain the steaks and transfer to a heated serving dish. Garnish with strips of chilli and serve with the salsa.

CALORIES PER SERVING: 200   FAT: 5G

Fight Fat, Fight Fatigue Diet and Cookbook

PORK AND APRICOT CASSEROLE

Pork has a real affinity with apricots. The sharpness of the fruit complements the taste and texture of the meat wonderfully.

4 x 200g/7oz lean pork loin chops or pork tenderloin steaks
1 onion, thinly sliced
2 yellow peppers, seeded and sliced
2 tsp medium curry powder
1 tbsp plain flour
250ml/8fl oz chicken stock
115g/4oz dried apricots
2 tbsp wholegrain mustard
Freshly ground black pepper
Chopped parsley for garnish

127

Trim any excess fat from the pork and brown lightly on both sides, without fat, in a heavy-bottomed casserole. Add the onion and yellow peppers to the pan and stir over a moderate heat for 5 minutes. Stir in the curry powder and flour. Add the stock, then the apricots and mustard. Cover and simmer for 25–30 minutes, until the lamb is tender. Add pepper to taste and serve garnished with parsley.

CALORIES PER SERVING: 370   FAT: 9.5G

Nutrition notes: *Pork is high in protein, B vitamins and minerals, though not as high in iron as other red meats like steak. However, it can be high in fat. This recipe uses lean pork which saves fat grams. The yellow peppers and dried apricots contain betacarotene, which has antioxidant properties.*

FILO SURPRISE PARCELS

Filo pastry is light and low in fat, so is a good substitute for ordinary pastry which is fat-loaded. Non-vegetarians could include chicken or prawns in one of the filo parcels.

12 sheets filo pastry, thawed if frozen
1 tsp olive oil

CHEESE FILLING:
75g/3oz feta cheese
124g/4oz pack cottage cheese with onion or chives
1 small egg, beaten

SPINACH FILLING:
75g/3oz frozen spinach, defrosted
1 tbsp grated low-fat hard cheese
Nutmeg to taste

VEGETABLE FILLING:
3 carrots, cut into small chunks
3 sticks celery, chopped
1 bunch spring onions, chopped
1 garlic clove, crushed
½ x 14oz/400g can artichokes, drained and halved
Vegetable stock cube

Preheat the oven to 200°C/400°F/Gas Mark 6. First, prepare the three fillings. In a bowl, mix the crumbled feta cheese, cottage cheese and beaten egg until smooth. In another bowl, mix the defrosted, drained spinach, cheese and nutmeg to taste. Add the stock cube to a pan of boiling water, add the carrots, celery, spring onion and garlic and simmer until crunchy. Drain and add the halved artichokes. Place filling in a third bowl and allow to cool.

Cut each sheet of filo pastry in half crossways to make two squares or rectangles. Lightly brush the pieces of pastry with oil, and place on top of each other at a 45-degree angle. Spoon a quarter of the cheese filling into the centre, gather the pastry up over the filling, and twist ends slightly to make a secure parcel. Repeat with three more from the first filling, then make four parcels with each of the other fillings. Place the parcels on a non-stick baking sheet and lightly brush all over with oil. Bake for 20 minutes, or until brown and crisp.

CALORIES PER PERSON (3 PARCELS): 200   FAT: 11G

Nutrition notes: *The fillings contain a variety of nutrients – calcium in the cheese, antioxidants in the spinach, and fibre and vitamins in the other vegetables. The garlic is a good addition too, as it lowers cholesterol.*

129

MEXICAN BAKED TROUT

4 trout, about 225g/8oz each
1 lemon
Small bunch fresh coriander
4 shallots, finely sliced
1 small yellow pepper, seeded and very finely chopped
1 small red pepper, seeded and finely chopped
2 green chillies, seeded and finely chopped
1 red chilli, seeded and finely chopped
1 tbsp lemon juice
1 tbsp white wine vinegar
2 tsp caster sugar
Salt and freshly ground black pepper
Extra coriander to garnish
Mixed salad leaves (lamb's lettuce, rocket, endive) to serve

Preheat the oven to 180°F/350°F/Gas Mark 4. Gut and wash the trout and pat dry with absorbent kitchen paper. Season and fill the cavities with freshly-squeezed lemon juice and a few coriander leaves. Put the fish, side by side, in a shallow ovenproof dish. Sprinkle over the shallots, peppers and chillies.

Mix the lemon juice, vinegar and sugar in a bowl and spoon over the trout. Season to taste (easy on the salt – you don't need much). Cover with foil and bake for 30 minutes or until the fish is tender. Transfer the fish to a warmed serving platter, top with the cooking juices and vegetables. Garnish with coriander and serve with salad leaves.

CALORIES PER SERVING: 250   FAT: 5.5G

PUDDINGS

FILO-TOPPED FRUIT PIE

900g/2lb Bramley or other cooking apples
6 tsp caster sugar
Grated rind of 1 lemon
1 tbsp lemon juice
85g/3oz sultanas
½ tsp ground cinnamon
4 large sheets filo pastry, thawed if frozen
2 tbsp low-fat spread, melted
Icing sugar, for dusting

131

Peel, core and dice the apples. Place them in a saucepan with caster sugar and lemon rind. Squeeze the lemon juice over the top, then bring to the boil. Stir well, lower the heat and simmer for 5 minutes, or until the apples soften. Stir in the sultanas and cinnamon. (You can use any soft, cooked fruit: try raspberries with redcurrants, blackberries with apple, or apricots with a dash of apricot brandy – yum!)

Spoon the fruity mixture into a 1.2 litre/2 pint pie dish and leave to cool. Heat the oven to 180°C/350°F/Gas Mark 4. Place a pie funnel or upturned egg cup in the centre of the fruit. Brush each sheet of filo with melted low-fat spread. Scrunch up loosely and place over the fruit to cover it completely. Bake for 20–30 minutes until golden. Dust the pie with icing sugar before serving.

CALORIES PER (LARGE!) SERVING: 290   FAT: 1G

SLIMMERS' PAVLOVA

MERINGUE:

175g/6oz soft light brown sugar
3 egg whites
1 tsp distilled malt vinegar
½ tsp vanilla essence

TOPPING:

1 tbsp icing sugar, sifted
300g/11oz 0% fat Greek yogurt
350g/12oz any fruit such as strawberries, raspberries, sliced peaches, plums, with a little kirsch, cassis or other liqueur to bring out the flavour

Preheat the oven to 160°C/325°F/Gas Mark 3. Draw a 20cm/8in circle on a sheet of non-stick baking paper, cut out and place on a baking sheet. Spread out the brown sugar on a second baking sheet and dry in the oven for about 8 minutes. Sieve to remove lumps.

Whisk the egg whites in a clean, grease-free bowl until stiff. Add half the soft brown sugar, 1 tablespoon at a time, whisking well. Add the vinegar and vanilla essence, then fold in the remaining sugar. Spoon the meringue onto the circle, leaving a central hollow. Bake for 45 minutes. Turn off the oven, open the door and leave the meringue until cold. Remove from the oven, carefully peel off the non-stick baking paper and transfer to a flat serving plate.

Stir most of the icing sugar into the Greek yogurt and spoon into the meringue centre. Top with fruit and dust with icing sugar.

CALORIES PER SERVING: 200   FAT: 0.5G

CHOCOLATE MOUSSE WITH RUM

A chocolate pud is the dream ending to most meals, but usually prohibited for slimmers. This one, however, is saintly!

500g/17oz carton low-fat fromage frais
150g/5oz 0% fat Greek yogurt
25g/1oz icing sugar
1 tbsp each low-fat drinking chocolate powder and cocoa powder
1 tsp vanilla essence
2 tbsp dark rum (optional)
2 medium egg whites
Grated dark chocolate for decoration

Combine the fromage frais and yogurt in a mixing bowl. Sift in the icing sugar, drinking chocolate and cocoa powder and mix well. Add the vanilla essence and rum, if using.

In a clean, dry bowl, whisk the egg whites until stiff. Using a metal spoon, fold the egg whites into the fromage frais mixture. Spoon the mixture into one large, or four small pots and chill in the refrigerator for 30 minutes. Just before serving, sprinkle with a little grated chocolate and serve with pieces of fresh fruit for dunking.

133

CALORIES PER SERVING: 150   FAT: 2G

Nutrition notes: *The fromage frais and Greek yogurt are both low in fat, and supply calcium; the egg whites contain protein. The rum is just alcohol (but you could use rum essence, if you are watching your booze intake), and the small amount of chocolate the recipe contains is just enough to give your taste buds a lift.*

DINNER PARTY GATEAU

This is a light and delicious dessert which would be very suitable for a special occasion such as a birthday, lunch or christening.

SPONGES:
A little low-fat spread
4 eggs, separated
75g/3oz granulated sugar
75g/3oz flour, sieved
1 tsp finely grated lemon rind

FILLING:
300g/11oz very low-fat soft cheese
450g/1lb raspberries
25g/1oz caster sugar
25g/1oz icing sugar

DECORATION:
A few raspberries or small fresh flowers
Egg white
A little caster sugar

Grease two 23cm/9 inch sandwich tins with a little low-fat spread and line with non-stick silicone paper. Cream the egg yolks with the sugar until very light, frothy and creamy. Whip the egg whites until stiff and stir into the yolks. Fold in the flour and lemon rind. Spread a quarter of the mixture in each sandwich tin, very thinly and carefully. Bake in a preheated 180°C/350°F/Gas Mark 4 oven for 5–7 minutes and turn out onto a flat surface to cool. Repeat the process so you have 4 thin sponges.

Fight Fat, Fight Fatigue Diet and Cookbook

Place one of the sponges on a cake stand or large plate. Spread over a layer of soft cheese. Arrange a third of the raspberries on top and sprinkle with a little sugar. Repeat the process with the remaining sponges. Sift the icing sugar over the top layer.

Decorate with a few raspberries dusted with sugar or, for a really special effect, paint small fresh flowers such as freesia or jasmine with egg white, then dredge with sugar and allow to dry for several hours, then place on top of the sponge.

SERVES: 6   CALORIES PER SERVING: 145   FAT: 7G

Nutrition notes: *The egg yolks contain fat, but they are also a good source of iron and vitamins A, B and D. The flour is a source of carbohydrate and the raspberries are rich in vitamin C. You could add extra fruits served separately to increase the vitamin and fibre content.*

135

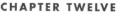

CHAPTER TWELVE

PICNICS AND BARBECUES

Healthy treats for the great outdoors

Eating al fresco is a fine way to get two of the things you really need for great health – good nutrition and plenty of fresh air. So why spoil it by overloading your system with fatty grub and calorific soft drinks? It's so easy to prepare delicious, portable, low-fat meals for your picnic, and stunning salads, meat, fish and vegetarian menus for your barbecue.

PICNICS

- Invest in a large coolbox and picnic hamper, and use real napkins, plates and tablecloths.
- Don't take any food which is going to spoil en route (i.e. sloppy sauces, mushy sarnies and limp salads) to your destination.
- Pack salads, rice and cold pasta dishes into large plastic bowls, and cover with cling film.
- If you are travelling by car, a folding table is handy. If not, pack the picnic into smaller containers so every member of the party can carry something.
- Once you arrive, search for a shady spot (not under a tree if it's stormy), check for ants' nests and similar hazards, and spread a groundsheet under your tablecloth to prevent damp patches spoiling your spread.

BARBECUES

- If you are using a charcoal-burning barbecue, remember that it can take an hour to heat properly.
- Invest in good quality fuel: lumpwood charcoal is cheaper and easier to light and burns hotter than pressed briquettes. However, the latter last longer, so are more economical. Once the flames are going and the coals have a grey ash all over the red glow, it is time to cook.
- Try not to have so much equipment to carry outside that the barbecue becomes a chore. One plate for each person, plus a couple of large platters of salad and vegetables (such as jacket potatoes) is enough.
- There is no need to slosh olive oil over everything – you can make delicious marinades using just a little oil plus other ingredients such as chilli sauce, red wine, stock, dry sherry, yogurt and lemon juice.

All recipes serve four, unless otherwise stated.

PITTA FILLINGS

Pitta breads are handy containers for other foods, so they're great for picnics – so long as you don't add fatty fillings!

8 large pittas
Watercress or salad leaves

CHICKEN CHILLI FILLING:

100g/4oz cooked chicken, shredded
2 tbsp tomato ketchup
1 tbsp malt vinegar
½ tsp chilli powder
1 green pepper, seeded and cut into strips
Salt and freshly ground black pepper

HAM AND SWEETCORN FILLING:

100g/4oz cooked ham, chopped
50g/2oz mushrooms, sliced
200g/7oz can sweetcorn kernels
2 tbsp fat-free French dressing

AVOCADO AND CHEESE FILLING:

1 large, ripe avocado
100g/4oz cottage cheese
1 tsp ground coriander
1 tsp lemon juice
Freshly ground black pepper

SALMON FILLING:

200g/7oz can pink salmon
1 tbsp low-fat mayonnaise
2 tsp lemon juice
1 tbsp chopped dill
Freshly ground black pepper

First, make the four fillings, mixing the ingredients and putting them into airtight containers. Split the pittas to make a pocket in each one, and pack separately. Four guests can each take two pittas, salad leaves and choose two of the fillings.

CALORIES PER SERVING (2 FILLED PITTAS): ABOUT 550   FAT: 14.5G

Nutrition notes: *Pitta bread is a good source of fibre and carbohydrate. The chicken, ham and salmon are high in protein, the sweetcorn provides vitamin A. Avocado also provides vitamin A and is a rich source of potassium. Watercress is a good source of iron.*

139

PICNIC TREATS

RICE AND FISH SALAD

225g/8oz long-grain brown rice
2 tsp paprika
225g/8oz smoked haddock (finnan haddie) fillet, cooked
1 small onion, finely chopped
50g/2oz seedless raisins
50g/2oz currants
50g/2oz cooked peas
50g/2oz canned sweetcorn kernels
2 small stalks celery, sliced
2 large tomatoes, sliced
10cm/4in cucumber, diced

DRESSING:
150g/5oz natural, unsweetened yogurt
75ml/3fl oz tomato juice
1 tsp each Worcestershire sauce and Dijon mustard
Freshly ground black pepper

Cook the rice in boiling, lightly salted water until tender (about 20 minutes). Drain and sprinkle with the paprika. Leave to cool.

Flake the fish, discarding any skin and bones. Mix with the onion, raisins, currants, peas, sweetcorn and celery. Press into a 1 litre/1¾ pint ring mould. Chill in the fridge for an hour, then cover with cling film to travel. Mix together the dressing ingredients and put in a screw-top jar. At the picnic, unmould the salad on to a large dish, fill the centre with tomato and cucumber, and pass around the dressing.

CALORIES PER PORTION: 330   FAT: 2.2G

Fight Fat, Fight Fatigue Diet and Cookbook

BURSTING BLOOMER

This is very popular with hungry men and children because it's so filling, and makes a welcome change from sandwiches.

1 small bloomer loaf
6 eggs, hard-boiled
40g/1½oz can dressed crab
100g/4oz can tuna in brine
2 tsp lemon juice
4 tbsp low-fat mayonnaise
2 tbsp tomato purée
Salt and ground black pepper
Lettuce and watercress leaves

Cut the loaf in half horizontally and, using a small knife and spoon, scoop out the bread from both pieces. Make about 75g/3oz into breadcrumbs.

Shell and finely chop the eggs and mix with the crab, flaked tuna, lemon juice, mayonnaise, tomato purée and breadcrumbs. Season. Line the bottom half of the bread shell with the salad leaves, pile in the filling, cover with the top half and press down. Wrap in foil and refrigerate for 2 hours before taking it on the picnic. To serve, cut the loaf into 2.5–5cm/1–2in thick slices.

CALORIES PER SERVING (⅙ LOAF): 230   FAT: 9.5G

Nutrition notes: *Bread contains calcium and carbohydrate, eggs are protein-packed and have iron in the yolks, and the tuna is also a good source of protein. However, the egg yolks do bump up the fat content.*

CHILLED CUCUMBER AND TARRAGON SOUP

The perfect picnic starter to serve on a hot summer's day by the river.

2 medium cucumbers, each about 20cm/8in long
150g/5oz onion
100g/4oz potato
900ml/30fl oz chicken stock
1 tbsp white wine vinegar
2 small sprigs freshly chopped tarragon or 1 tsp dried tarragon
A little salt and white pepper

TO SERVE:
4 tbsp natural low-fat yogurt
Curled strips of cucumber peel
Tiny sprigs of fresh tarragon

Peel the cucumbers, saving some peel to cut into circle strips for garnish. Cut in half lengthwise, scoop out the seeds and chop the flesh into chunks. Peel and chop the onion and potato and put them into a pan with the chicken stock and cucumber chunks. Add vinegar and tarragon and simmer, uncovered, for 20 minutes. Liquidize in a blender and season to taste. Chill and put in a Thermos flask to take to the picnic. Serve in cups, garnished with yogurt, cucumber peel and fresh tarragon.

CALORIES PER PERSON: 75   FAT: NEG.

Nutrition notes: *This refreshing soup is mildly diuretic (water-chasing), thanks to the cucumber, and also supplies calcium (in the yogurt). Tarragon is a herb which is good for the digestion, and was used in ancient times to cure toothache.*

Fight Fat, Fight Fatigue Diet and Cookbook

BARBECUE DISHES

PORK AND LIME KEBABS

675g/1½lb pork fillet cut into bite-sized cubes
3 limes, sliced
4 small bananas

MARINADE:
4 tbsp dark rum
2 tsp grated lime rind
1 tbsp each lime juice and grated ginger
3 cloves garlic, crushed
2 tsp brown sugar
Seasoning

143

Place the pork in a shallow dish. Combine all the marinade ingredients and pour over the meat. Leave for 1 hour, or overnight.

Thread the meat pieces onto skewers, alternating with folded slices of lime. Cook for 15–20 minutes, turning and brushing with the marinade to keep moist. Remove a small strip of skin from each banana, brush with the marinade, and place, open-side down on the barbecue. Cook for 1 minute, turn over and cook for 2 minutes. Serve with the kebabs.

CALORIES PER SERVING: 340   FAT: 10G

Nutrition notes: *Pork is high in protein, B vitamins and minerals. Limes contain vitamin C, and bananas potassium and carbohydrate. Garlic helps lower cholesterol. The rum and sugar are not particularly wicked, and very tasty.*

CAJUN CHICKEN WITH SALSA

Chicken can often be bland-tasting, but this spicy marinade and salsa certainly peps it up without adding fat.

4 boneless chicken breasts
1 tbsp oil
½ small onion, very finely chopped
1 garlic clove, finely chopped

CAJUN SPICE MIXTURE:

2 tsp paprika
1 tsp each mustard powder, cayenne pepper, ground cumin, dried thyme, dried oregano
½ tsp each ground black pepper and salt

SALSA:

2 medium tomatoes
Small bunch coriander
200g/7oz sweetcorn kernels
1 small red onion, finely chopped
1 red chilli, finely chopped
2 tbsp lime or lemon juice

Remove the skin from the chicken breasts and make deep diagonal slashes in the meat. Brush each with a very little oil. Pound the onion and garlic to a paste in a pestle and mortar or with the back of a spoon. Transfer to a bowl and mix in the spices. Rub over the chicken breasts, then chill for an hour. Dice the tomatoes finely, chop the fresh coriander and place in a bowl with the sweetcorn, red onion, chilli and lime or lemon juice.

Place the chicken on a prepared barbecue and cook for 20 minutes (or until juices run clear when you pierce the thickest part of the breast), turning once. Serve with the salsa.

CALORIES PER SERVING: 130   FAT: 1.5G

Nutrition notes: *The mixture of herbs and spices benefits the circulation and helps fight infection, the garlic helps lower cholesterol, and the lime or lemon juice adds some vitamin C.*

145

STEAKS IN COGNAC WITH FROMAGE FRAIS

This is a delicious, luxury meal that will make your barbie that little bit special.

4 fillet steaks, about 175g/6oz each
4 tbsp low-fat fromage frais

COGNAC MARINADE:

1 tbsp olive oil
4 tbsp cognac
1 tsp freshly ground black pepper
1 tbsp each chopped fresh chives and fresh thyme
Parsley or watercress for garnish

146

Place the steaks in a shallow dish. Combine the marinade ingredients and pour over. Leave in the refrigerator overnight. Place the steak on the grill rack, cook for 5–6 minutes each side, brushing frequently with the marinade. Serve each steak topped with a tablespoon of fromage frais and chopped parsley or watercress sprigs.

CALORIES PER SERVING: 160   FAT: 10G

Nutrition notes: *Steak is an excellent source of iron and protein, and the fromage frais provides calcium. Most of the alcohol from the cognac will evaporate with cooking, so this luscious dish won't make you drunk!*

CHINESE SALAD WITH GINGER

The dressing turns this simple salad into a treat. It goes very well with grilled chicken or fish.

50g/2oz beansprouts
50g/2oz grated carrot
50g/2oz seeded and chopped green and red pepper
2 sticks celery
50g/2oz sliced water chestnuts
Crisp iceberg lettuce or Chinese leaves

DRESSING:
2 tbsp light soy sauce
2 tbsp sesame oil
2 tbsp dry sherry
½ tsp Chinese five spice powder
1 tsp grated fresh ginger
½ garlic clove, crushed

Put the dressing ingredients into a screw-topped jar. Shake well and leave for an hour so that the flavours blend. Combine the salad ingredients in a large bowl, give the dressing a shake, and pour over. Toss well and serve in a bed of iceberg lettuce or Chinese leaves.

CALORIES PER SERVING: 90   FAT: 7G

Nutrition notes: *Ginger is renowned as a stimulant, and many people swear by it as a cold cure. The salad contains vitamin A and fibre in the carrot, and vitamin C and fibre in the red pepper. The sesame seed oil in the dressing contains the healthy monounsaturated and polyunsaturated types of oil, beneficial for the heart and circulation.*

Picnics and Barbecues

FRUITY KEBABS

Hot, grilled fruit is absolutely luscious-tasting, and so good for slimmers. Enjoy!

1 small pineapple, peeled and cut into chunks
3 firm nectarines or peaches, halved, stoned and cut into thick slices
225g/8oz strawberries
3 kiwi fruit, cut into quarters
2 red apples, quartered, cored and cut into thick slices
2 tsp caster sugar
Low-fat Greek yogurt, to serve

Thread the pieces of fruit onto skewers, sprinkle with a little sugar and place on the grill rack of the barbecue. Grill, turning occasionally, for about 5–7 minutes until warm and sticky! Serve each kebab with 1 tablespoon of low-fat Greek yogurt.

CALORIES PER SERVING: 160   FAT: 0.6G

Nutrition notes: *Cooking fruit destroys some nutrients, but this is still a very good way of getting at least one of your 'five portions of fruit and vegetables a day' which the government recommends. Kiwi fruit, strawberries and apples provide vitamin C. Pineapple is good for aiding digestion and it contains manganese and potassium, as well as vitamin C.*

RESOURCES

Food for thought

Here are some reading suggestions and contacts to help you increase your knowledge about healthy eating and have more fun in the kitchen.

Reading

You will also enjoy the two companion books in the Sun Slimmer series:

- *Energy Makeover* by Sally Ann Voak and Nicki Waterman
- *Firm Up All Over* by Nicki Waterman

Recipe websites

www.kelloggs.co.uk
Healthy recipe ideas and plenty of nutritional information. Worth a browse for breakfast-lovers, and a great help to slimmers.

www.nestle.co.uk
Recipes for everyday meals and dinner parties. The ones using Waistline low-fat dressings are particularly useful.

www.quorn.com
Lots of brilliant recipes using Quorn, the no-meat alternative made from tiny mushrooms (no GM ingredients).

www.pridevalley.com
Regularly updated seasonal recipes using pitta bread and tortilla wraps, which make a good alternative to sandwiches for lunch.

Contacts

British Dietetic Association, 5th Floor, Charles House, 148/9 Great Charles Street, Queensway, Birmingham, B3 3HT **www.bda.uk.com**

British Nutrition Foundation, High Holborn House, 52–54 High Holborn, London WC1 6RQ **www.nutrition.org.uk**

Dieticians in Sport and Exercise Nutrition, PO Box 22360, London W13 9FL

Food Standards Agency, Room 621, Hannibal House, PO Box 30080, Elephant and Castle, London SE1 6YA **www.foodstandards.gov.uk**

FSA Publications, PO Box 369, Hayes, Middlesex, UB3 IUT (free booklets include Food Safety, Understanding Food Labels, Healthy Eating)

The Nutrition Society, 10 Cambridge Court, 210 Shepherds Bush Road, London W6 7NJ **www.nutsoc.org.uk**

The Vegetarian Society, Parkdale, Dunham Road, Altrincham, Cheshire, WA14 4QG **www.vegsoc.org**

The Vegan Society, 7 Battle Road, St. Leonards-on-Sea, East Sussex, TN37 7AA **www.vegansociety.com**

Sally Ann Voak, PO Box 618, Coulsdon, Surrey CR5 IRU

PLEASE NOTE: CONTACT DETAILS CORRECT AT TIME OF GOING TO PRESS.

INDEX

152